Katrin Döhnel

Theory of Mind, Emotion, and the Brain

Katrin Döhnel

Theory of Mind, Emotion, and the Brain

Brain Regions involved in Intention-Based Emotion Attribution

Südwestdeutscher Verlag für Hochschulschriften

Imprint
Any brand names and product names mentioned in this book are subject to trademark, brand or patent protection and are trademarks or registered trademarks of their respective holders. The use of brand names, product names, common names, trade names, product descriptions etc. even without a particular marking in this work is in no way to be construed to mean that such names may be regarded as unrestricted in respect of trademark and brand protection legislation and could thus be used by anyone.

Publisher:
Südwestdeutscher Verlag für Hochschulschriften
is a trademark of
Dodo Books Indian Ocean Ltd., member of the OmniScriptum S.R.L Publishing group
str. A.Russo 15, of. 61, Chisinau-2068, Republic of Moldova Europe
Printed at: see last page
ISBN: 978-3-8381-2515-2

Zugl. / Approved by: München, LMU, Diss., 2009

Copyright © Katrin Döhnel
Copyright © 2011 Dodo Books Indian Ocean Ltd., member of the OmniScriptum S.R.L Publishing group

ACKNOWLEDGEMENTS

The aim of this thesis is to explore the neural network involved in intention-based emotion attribution. I want to thank all those people who supported me in the completion of this thesis. First of all I want to thank my supervisors Professor Beate Sodian and Professor Göran Hajak for their continuous and valuable support particularly with respect to providing both the theoretical and material ground throughout all stages of this thesis. Furthermore, I am much obliged to Monika Sommer and Jörg Meinhardt who always support me and let me participate in their scientific experiences. Many thanks also to my colleagues at the Clinical Neuroscience Centre for Emotions and Social Cognition: Kerstin Eichenmüller, Katrin Arnold, Christoph Rothmayr, Tobias Schuwerk, and Johannes Schwerdtner. I also want to thank all participants for taking part in the experiments. I am also much obliged to my family who always encourage and support me.

CONTENTS

General Introduction 7

1. Introduction
Study I – Emotions inferred from intention-outcome-relations 9

1.1 Developmental findings on the processing of intention-outcome relations 9

1.2 Neuroimaging findings on Theory of Mind 15

    1.2.1 False belief reasoning 15

    1.2.2 Intention attribution 20

    1.2.3 Emotion attribution 23

1.3 Summary and research question 25

2. Methods
Study I – Emotions inferred from intention-outcome-relations 26

2.1 Participants 26

2.2 Task and material 26

2.3 Experimental procedure 28

2.4 Statistical analysis of the behavioural data 31

2.5 Imaging and image preprocessing 31

2.6 Statistical analysis of the images 32

3. Results
Study I – Emotions inferred from intention-outcome-relations 33

3.1 Behavioural findings 33

3.2 Neuroimaging findings 37

4. Discussion
Study I – Emotions inferred from intention-outcome-relations 43

4.1 Behavioural findings 43
4.2 Neuroimaging findings 44
    4.2.1 Activity increase in the medial pre-SMA 44
    4.2.2 Activity increase in the dorsolateral prefrontal cortex 47
    4.2.3 Activity increase in the ventrolateral prefrontal cortex 50
    4.2.4 Activity decrease in the orbital part of the paracingulate cortex 50
4.3 Summary 52

5. Introduction
Study II – Emotions inferred from the integration of immoral intentions into intention-outcome-relations 54

5.1 The happy victimizer phenomenon 54
5.2 Neuroimaging findings on the processing of transgression scenarios 61
5.3 Summary and research question 63

6. Methods
Study II – Emotions inferred from the integration of immoral intentions into intention-outcome-relations 64

6.1 Participants 64
6.2 Task and material 64
6.3 Experimental procedure 69
6.4 Statistical analysis of the behavioural data 69
6.5 Imaging and image preprocessing 69
6.6 Statistical analysis of the images 70

7. Results
Study II – Emotions inferred from the integration of immoral intentions into intention-outcome-relations 73

7.1 Behavioural findings 73
7.2 Neuroimaging findings 83

8. Discussion

Study II – Emotions inferred from the integration of immoral intentions into intention-outcome-relations 91

    4.1 Behavioural findings 91

    4.2 Neuroimaging findings 92

    4.3 Summary 94

9. General Discussion and Perspectives 95

10. Summary 97

11. References 99

Appendix A: Index of figures and tables 108
Appendix B: Example of the rating material 112

GENERAL INTRODUCTION

The ability to infer another person's emotions from his or her intention is closely developed around the ability to understand false beliefs, the key Theory of Mind (ToM) ability. False belief understanding is acquired at the age of 4- to 5-years and is supposed to be an indicator of representational understanding (for reviews on ToM in developmental psychology see Astington, 1993; Perner, 1991b; Sodian & Thoermer, 2006; Wellman, 1990; Wellman, Cross, & Watson, 2001). By the age of 2½ to 4 years, children begin to attribute emotions based on processing simple intention-outcome-relations. Inferring emotions from simple intention-outcome-relations is assumed to not require representational operations (Astington, 1999a; Astington, 2001b; Baird & Astington, 2005; Perner, 1991a). From the age of six to seven years, children begin to properly integrate others' immoral intentions into intention-outcome relations. Developmental evidence indicates that the ability to infer emotions from other's immoral intentions is based on the development of representational understanding (Baird & Astington, 2004; Sokol, 2004; Sokol & Chandler, 2004; Sokol, Chandler, & Jones, 2004). This thesis is the first that investigates the neural correlates associated with inferring emotions based on mental states such as intentions. By identifying the brain regions associated with intention-based emotion attribution, functional neuroimaging can help clarify whether intention-based emotion attribution is associated with common or distinct neural networks relative to false belief understanding.

Because false belief processing is the key ToM ability, until now the majority of neuroimaging studies have concentrated on exploring the neural correlates associated with false belief understanding (for reviews on neuroimaging evidence on false belief understanding see Amodio & Frith, 2006; Frith & Frith, 2006; Frith & Frith, 2003; Gallagher & Frith, 2003; Saxe, 2006; Saxe & Baron-Cohen, 2006; Saxe, Carey, & Kanwisher, 2004). Other neuroimaging studies have explored the attribution of mental states such as intentions (Brunet, Sarfati, Hardy-Bayle, & Decety, 2000; Castelli, Frith, Happe, & Frith, 2002; Gobbini, Koralek, Bryan, Montgomery, & Haxby, 2007; Martin & Weisberg, 2003; Schultz, 2005; Tavares, Lawrence, & Barnard, 2008; Walter et al., 2004), or emotions (Baron-Cohen et al., 1999; Heberlein, Adolphs, Tranel, & Damasio, 2004; Hynes, Baird, & Grafton, 2006; Ochsner et al., 2004; Ruby & Decety, 2004; Schulte-Ruther, Markowitsch, Fink, & Piefke, 2007; Wicker, Perrett, Baron-Cohen, & Decety, 2003). These studies, however, have explored mental state attribution based on physical cues. A full ToM understanding, however, requires the prediction and explanation of others' behaviour, including their emotional reactions, independent of physical cues, that is, solely on inferring behaviour from mental cues. This criterion is fulfilled for emotion attribution based on mental states such as intentions.

To explore intention-based emotion attribution in healthy adults, two experiments were conducted. In both experiments nonverbal stories with verbal vignettes were presented, which were adopted from developmental studies on intention-based emotion attribution (Yuill, Perner, Pearson, Peerbhoy, & van den Ende, 1996). The nonverbal material was held equivalent across the experimental conditions, which only differed in their verbal vignettes. Experiment 1 concentrates on emotion attribution based on processing simple intention-outcome-relations, in which an actor's intention either matched or mismatched the outcome situation. By realizing a 2 by 2 factorial design, experiment 2 investigates emotion attribution based on integrating an actor's immoral intention into intention-outcome-relations. Here, the factor intention varied on whether the protagonist held a neutral or immoral intention. Analogous to experiment 1 the factor 'intention-outcome-relation' in experiment 2 varied on whether the protagonist's intention matched or mismatched the outcome situation. In both experiments, besides emotion attribution conditions, a non-mental control condition was used that solely described physical processes. The functional magnetic resonance imaging (fMRI) analysis focussed on the emotion attribution cue.

In chapter 1 the experiment 1 is introduced, followed by a method, result, and discussion part (chapters 2 to 4). In chapter 5 the experiment 2 is introduced, followed by a method, result, and discussion part (chapters 6 to 8). Further, the thesis contains a general discussion and perspectives on future research (chapter 9). Finally, the thesis is concluded with a summary (chapter 10).

1. INTRODUCTION

STUDY I
EMOTIONS INFERRED FROM INTENTION-OUTCOME-RELATIONS

The aim of experiment one is to investigate the neural correlates associated with the processing of emotions inferred from intention-outcome-relations. This ability is developed shortly before the ability to understand false beliefs, that is, between 2½ and 4 years of age. Developmental findings on the processing of intention-outcome-relations are summarized in chapter 1.1, followed by a review of the neural network involved in Theory of Mind (chapter 1.2). Finally, the introduction of experiment one concludes with a summary and a deduction of the research question (chapter 1.3).

1.1 Developmental findings on the processing of intention-outcome relations

By the age of 2½ to 4 years children judge a person holding a neutral intention as feeling happy when a desired goal is fulfilled and as feeling sad when the desired goal is not fulfilled (Astington, 1999a; Feinfield, Lee, Flavell, Green, & Flavell, 1999; Hadwin & Perner, 1991; Lagattuta, 2005; Stein & Levine, 1989; Wellman & Banerjee, 1991; Wellman & Woolley, 1990; Yuill, 1984; Yuill et al., 1996). However, 2½ - to 4-years-olds' understanding of mental states is a rather limited one. They have not yet acquired the concept that mental states belong to persons, independent of situations. Rather, they process others' mental states as being (objectively) bound to situations than being (subjectively) associated with a person. Developmental psychologists assume that when 2½- to 4-years-old attribute emotions based on intention-outcome situations, they rely on a matching strategy, that is, they infer an actor's emotion by matching the factual outcome situation with the hypothetical 'intended situation' (Astington, 1999a; Astington, 2001b; Baird & Astington, 2005; Perner, 1991a). Specifically, in the case where an actor's 'intended situation' matches the outcome situation, the actor is judged to feel good (e.g. intended situation: Max wants to throw the ball to Anna; outcome situation: Max throws the ball to Anna). In contrast, when there is a mismatch between the 'intended situation' and the outcome situation, the actor is judged to feel sad (e.g. intended situation: Max wants to throw the ball to Anna; outcome situation: Max throws the ball to Tim).

There is much empirical evidence which underpins the assumption that 2½- to 4-year-olds' ability for emotion attribution is limited to an intention-outcome-matching strategy. First, Yuill (1984) investigated whether young children could integrate an actor's immoral intention into intention-outcome-relations. The author presented picture stories that depicted an actor's intention, an action, and an outcome. The actor's intention varied on the dimensions neutral (e.g., [an actor] wants to throw the ball to person A) and immoral (e.g., [an actor] wants to hit person A with the ball). The outcome either matched (e.g., neutral intention: person A catches the ball; immoral intention: person A is hit by the ball), or mismatched the actor's intention. In cases of an intention-outcome mismatch, the actor's intention either mismatched the outcome with respect to the recipient (mismatch-recipient; neutral intention: person B [instead of person A] catches the ball; immoral intention: person B [instead of person A] is hit by the ball), or with respect to the value of the actor's intention (mismatch-value; neutral intention: person A is hit by the ball [instead of catching the ball]; immoral intention: person A catches the ball [instead of being hit by the ball]). Children had to judge the actor's satisfaction and had to perform morality judgements. With respect to satisfaction judgements, the author assumed that for both neutral and immoral intentions, children would attribute positive emotions to an actor who fulfilled its intention. In contrast, an actor whose intention did not match the intended outcome was supposed to be judged to feel sad. With respect to morality judgements, Yuill (1984) assumed that when reasoning about moral values, a wrongdoer had to be judged worse than a 'neutral' actor regardless of the outcome. Regarding satisfaction judgments, 3-year-olds, as did 5- and 7-year-olds, appropriately judged an actor holding a neutral intention as more satisfied in situations were its neutral intention matches the outcome compared to situations where the outcome mismatches the actor's intention. Interestingly, 3-years-olds did not show that distinction for immoral intentions. They judged an actor who fulfilled his or her immoral intention feeling as sad as an actor whose immoral intention was not fulfilled. With respect to morality judgements, 5- and 7-year-olds appropriately judged a wrongdoer worse than an actor holding a neutral intention, irrespective of the outcome situation. Interestingly, 3-year-olds' morality judgements were related to the outcome scenario. For example, victimizers who accidentally caused a neutral outcome were not judged worse than neutral actors who accidentally caused a negative outcome. Moreover, neutral actors causing harm accidentally were judged worse than neutral actors causing no harm. Furthermore, wrongdoers who accidentally caused a neutral outcome were judged to be better than wrongdoers who accidentally hurt the wrong recipient. The results provide evidence that 3-year-olds' ability to integrate an actor's immoral intention into the processing of intention-outcome-relations are primarily based on processing an intention in relation to outcome cues (outcome orientation) rather than processing an intention as being a person's mental state, independent of the outcome.

These results were confirmed by another study (Yuill et al., 1996) that presented stories similar to the stories given in the study of Yuill (1984). In this study, 3-year-olds also gave outcome-oriented responses to wrongdoers, that is, wrongdoers were judged to feel sad, regardless of whether its immoral intention resulted in goal attainment or not. Moreover, Yuill et al. (1996) showed a developmental trend with respect to intention-based emotion attribution from taking an objective stance in 3-year-olds (children's emotion attribution responses referred to the outcome) to taking a subjective stance in 5- to 7-year-olds (children's emotion attribution responses referred to the actor's intention) to taking a moral stance in 10-year-olds (children's emotion attribution responses contained moral considerations; for a review on the literature investigating young children's happy victimizer patterns see chapter 5.1). Taking a subjective stance in 5- to 7-year-olds resulted in the attribution of positive emotions to a wrongdoer, that is, emotion judgements were oriented towards goal attainment, irrespective of moral transgression. Taking a moral stance in 10-year-olds were based on mixed emotion patterns, that is, feeling both bad at the moral transgression and good at having attained the desired goal. In another experiment, the authors reasoned that as soon as children can take a subjective stance in addition to an objective stance they can learn to integrate both stances. The authors assumed that this should result in the ability to develop a moral stance, which is supposed to be based on both subjective (goal attainment) and objective considerations (moral transgression). The authors assumed that not before the age of five children should be able to flexibly switch between stances, because before age five children are supposed to be only capable of the objective stance. To test these assumptions, the authors manipulated different stances by asking children morally (e.g., 'Was that a good or bad thing for [the actor] to do?') or personally salient questions (e.g., 'Was that what [the actor] wanted to happen or not what [the actor] wanted to happen?') before they asked children the emotion attribution questions based on the intention-outcome stories described above. Interestingly, while 5-year-olds' judgements varied by the stance manipulations, 3-year-olds' judgements did not. That is, while 5-year-olds judged a wrongdoer whose immoral goal was attained less happy in the moral salience condition than in the personal salience conditions, 3-year-olds did not show such an effect. These results suggest that 3-year-olds' ability to process mental states such as intentions are yet bound to situations rather than to persons since they are not capable to switch between a subjective and a moral stance.

A second argument for the assumption that 2½- to 4-year-olds attribute emotion by an intention-outcome-matching strategy comes from empirical evidence that 3- to 4-years-olds have difficulties in dealing with belief-based emotion attribution tasks (Hadwin & Perner, 1991; Wellman & Banerjee, 1991). For example, Hadwin & Perner (1991) explored whether 3- to 4-year-olds would be able to reason about emotions such as happiness and surprise. While happiness is more the consequence of intention-outcome-relations, surprise is rather a consequence of belief-outcome-relations. Similar to the stories presented in Yuill (1984), children had to attribute emotions to a character based on either intention-outcome-relations (e.g., intention: [an actor] wants to throw the ball to Person A; outcome match: Person A catches the ball; outcome mismatch: Person B catches the ball) or based on belief-outcome-relations (e.g., belief: [an actor] believes that person A has the ball; belief-outcome match (true belief): person A has the ball; belief-outcome mismatch (false belief): person B has the ball). With respect to the intention-outcome stories, the authors reasoned that an actor should be judged to feel happy in cases of goal attainment, and to feel unhappy in cases of missing a desired goal. Regarding the belief-outcome scenarios, an actor should be judged to feel surprised in situations where his or her belief mismatches the outcome. In contrast, the character should be judged as not being surprised in cases where the belief matches the outcome. Three- to four-year-olds managed to attribute happiness to the actor in situations where a desired outcome was reached and unhappiness in stories where the desire was unfulfilled. Interestingly, 3- to 4-year-olds performed at chance in judging a character as not being surprised in belief-outcome-match stories and as being surprised in belief-outcome-mismatch trials.

These results were confirmed in another study on belief-based emotion attribution (Wellman & Banerjee, 1991). The authors presented belief-desire-outcome stories to 3-year-olds and explored their ability to attribute to an actor the more desire-based emotion happiness and the more belief-based emotion surprise. For example, one situation type depicted a protagonist who wants sunshine (desire), thinks that it will rain (belief), and it finally rains (outcome). This situation was designed as depicting a desire that mismatched the outcome and a belief that matched the outcome; hence unhappiness and no surprise should be attributed. Another story type depicted an actor who, for example, wants a goldfish (desire), thinks that he will get a goldfish (belief), and finally obtains a cow (outcome). Here, the correct emotion pattern would be unhappiness with respect to a desire that mismatches the outcome, and surprise with respect to a belief-outcome-mismatch. A third scenario required happiness judgements with respect to a desire that matches the outcome and surprise judgements based on belief-outcome-mismatch: for example, a character wants grape juice (desire), thinks that he will get milk (belief), and finally gets grape juice (outcome). Regarding reasoning about desire-outcome-relations, 3-year-olds correctly attributed happiness to desire match situations and unhappiness to desire mismatch situations. However, they showed less competence in correctly attributing the belief-dependent emotion surprise. These findings were further supported by another experiment. Wellman & Banerjee (1991) reasoned whether an emotion explanation method would be a more sensitive instrument to measure 3-year-olds' ability in belief-based emotion attribution. They presented the same stories as described above, but children did not need to infer the appropriate emotion. Instead, the appropriate emotion was presented to the child after story presentation. The child was then asked to explain why the actor was feeling this way. Responses were categorized into desire and belief-based responses. Interestingly, even with a more sensitive measure, the 3-year-olds' lack in belief-based emotion attribution remained. Three-year-olds' responses did not differentiate with respect to the more desire-based emotion happiness and the more belief-based emotion surprise. Furthermore, they showed a bias for desire-based responses since for both happiness and surprise they gave more desire-based responses. In addition, belief-based responses were rarely given.

A third argument for the assumption that 2½- to 4-year-olds attribute emotion based on an intention-outcome-matching strategy comes from empirical evidence that 3- to 4-year-olds show less competence in reasoning about intentions in cases where intentions are not directly related to a situation (Feinfield et al., 1999; Schult, 2002). Feinfield et al. (1999) presented stories to 3-year-olds in which an actor's intention (e.g., going to the football stadium for their mother's sake) mismatched both that actor's desire (e.g., going to the mountains for their own sake) and the desired outcome (e.g., bus gets lost and ends up at the mountains). The authors assumed that in order to identify the actor's intention, the children had to process the intention independent of both the desire and the desired outcome. The authors reasoned that in such scenarios, intention processing would require taking a subjective stance rather than an objective stance. Three-year-olds showed competence in reasoning about the actor's desire ('Where does [the actor] like to go?'; correct answer: 'to the mountains'). Compared to 4-year-olds, however, 3-year-olds showed less competence in reasoning about the actor's intention ('Where did [the actor] try do go?'; 'Where did [the actor] think he was going to go?'; correct answer: 'to the football stadium'). As a methodological limitation, Astington (2001) points out that in Feinfield et al.'s (1999) study, intentions could have been inferred by a matching-strategy as well, because desires and intention were not causally linked to the same outcome. The character's intention was linked to the goal to go the football stadium in order to follow his mother's wishes. His desire, however, was linked to a different goal, that is, to go to the mountains. Therefore, Astington (2001) argues that although the intention mismatches the desired goal, it matches the intended goal. In order to explore whether intentions are understood independent of the outcome, a better way to distinguish intentions and desire would be to present scenarios where both intentions and desires are related to the same goal, whereas there is a match between desire and goal and a mismatch between intention and that goal. Schult (2002) realized such scenarios by presenting 4-, 5-, 7-year-olds and adults picture stories in which an actor's desire was fulfilled, however, it was fulfilled in an unintended fashion (e.g., desire: Becky wants to have a doll; intention: Becky plans to buy herself that doll; outcome (desire fulfilled / intention unfulfilled): Becky's mother gave her the doll). While 5-, 7-year-olds and adults could distinguish between the actor's desire ('Did Becky get what she wanted?'; correct answer: 'yes') and the actor's intention ('Did Becky do what she planned to do?'; correct answer: 'no'), 4-year-olds could correctly answer the desire question, but, performed at chance with respect to the intention question.

A fourth argument for the assumption that 2½- to 4-year-olds attribute emotion by an intention-outcome-matching strategy comes from empirical evidence which indicates that when the matching strategy between the intention and the outcome is not made salient, 3-year-olds show a lack in competence in reasoning about the character's intention (Astington, 1999a; Baird & Moses, 2002). For example, Astington (1999) contrasted an implicit intention-outcome condition (e.g., 'Ernie has some bread. He takes it outside. He throws crumbs down. The birds pick them up.') with an unintended, accidental, condition (e.g., 'Bert's got some bread too. He walks along eating it. Some crumbs fall behind him. The birds pick them up.'), and with an explicit intention-outcome control story where intention and outcome were made salient. Three types of test questions were asked. The 'try question' required the children to reason about an intention-in action (Searle, 1983), that is, an intention that an actor is actually carrying out (e.g., 'Here's Ernie, and here's Bert. Which guy tried to get the birds to eat crumbs?'; correct answer: 'Ernie') The authors reasoned that to answer this question appropriately, the intention has to be inferred from situational variables. The 'meant question' targeted on the prior-intention (Searle, 1983), that is, an intention that an actor is actually not carrying out, but that he is going to carry out (e.g., 'Here's Ernie, and here's Bert. Which guy meant the birds to eat the crumbs?'; correct answer: 'Ernie'). Astington (1999) reasoned that prior-intentions cannot be directly inferred from situational cues, but have to be processed independent of the reality state. Group differences were only found for the 'meant question' that was supposed to require reasoning about prior-intentions. Three-year-olds were less likely to give appropriate answers than 4- and 5-year-olds. Based on these results, Astington (1999) assumes that 3-year-olds competence in intention-based emotion attribution is rather based on matching different situations than on understanding the subjective nature of a mental state. Further evidence that children beyond 5 years of age have difficulties in processing intentions independent of reality cues comes from a recent study (Baird & Moses, 2002). The authors presented characters that had different desires (e.g., to be home for dinner vs. to be healthy and strong), but performed the same action (e.g., running). Four- and five-year-olds were asked for the character's intention (e.g., to get somewhere fast vs. to get some exercise). While 5-year-olds correctly attributed different intentions despite the same actions, 4-year-olds performed at chance with respect to intention attribution.

In sum, there is strong evidence that 2½- to 4-year-olds perform intention-based emotion attribution tasks based on an objective stance, that is, by processing an intention in relation to an outcome situation rather than based on a subjective stance, that is, by processing an intention independent of reality cues (Astington, 1999a; Astington, 2001b; Baird & Astington, 2005; Perner, 1991a). Although 2½- to 4-year-olds appropriately attribute emotions based on a neutral intention, they show less competence in tasks where a subjective stance is supposed to be more effective, that is, they show inappropriate emotion responses for immoral intentions (Yuill, 1984; Yuill et al.,

1996), do not successfully handle belief-based emotion attribution tasks (Hadwin & Perner, 1991; Wellman & Banerjee, 1991), and show less competence in reasoning about intentions in cases where intentions are not directly related to a situation (Feinfield et al., 1999; Schult, 2002). Finally, they show less competence when the intention-outcome-relation is not made salient (Astington, 1999a; Baird & Moses, 2002). The ability to attribute emotions based on intention-outcome-relations shortly precedes the acquirement of false belief reasoning. Therefore, developmental findings suggest distinct rather than common neural networks, since there seems to be a change in mental state understanding from taking an objective stance in 2½- to 4-year-olds to taking a subjective stance above age 4. However, direct evidence is still lacking. The following chapters review neuroimaging findings on the ToM network.

1.2 Neuroimaging findings on Theory of Mind

Neuroimaging can help address the question of whether there are distinct or common neuronal networks associated with false belief understanding and intention-based emotion attribution. To date, there are many neuroimaging studies on false belief understanding and on inferring mental states from physical cues, an ability that develops much earlier than false belief understanding and intention-based emotion attribution. This is the first study that investigates the functional basis of emotion attribution based on intention-outcome-relations, an ability that shortly precedes the development of false belief understanding. Chapter 1.2 starts by reviewing neuroimaging findings on false belief reasoning (chapter 1.2.1), followed by neuroimaging evidence on intention attribution (chapter 1.2.2) and emotion attribution (chapter 1.2.3).

1.2.1 False belief reasoning

The false belief task originally designed by Wimmer & Perner (1983) is the critical test to assess whether a person has a Theory of Mind (ToM), since it requires one to understand that people act according to their beliefs, independent of the state of reality. Critically, false belief reasoning is based on understanding that a person's false representation about reality is believed to be a true representation about reality by that person. In order to differentiate these two mental representations of reality, the true belief I hold and the false belief the other holds, one is supposed to require the ability to represent mental states independent of reality (Perner, 1991b; Sodian & Thoermer, 2006).

Initially, ToM research in neuroimaging was inspired by research on autism (Baron-Cohen, Leslie, & Frith, 1985). It was robustly found that autistic children are significantly more likely to fail the false belief task than normally developing children (for reviews see Hill & Frith, 2003; Sodian, 2005). Based on this finding, it was argued that reasoning about false beliefs should be subserved by a brain region specifically associated with ToM (Frith & Frith, 1999). Since the false belief task is the critical test for having a ToM, most neuroimaging studies have concentrated on exploring the neural network associated with false belief reasoning. To explore the functional basis associated with false belief understanding, neuroscientist defined criteria a neural network should meet in order to be a candidate network for subserving ToM (Perner, Aichhorn, Kronbichler, Staffen, & Ladurner, 2006; Saxe et al., 2004; Stone & Gerrans, 2006). The functional circuitry involved in ToM should not only be necessary for processing ToM, but it should also be specialized for ToM. In other words, (1) the ToM network should respond to belief reasoning in general, both true and false beliefs, (2) the ToM network should show a significantly stronger response to mental states that require representation about mental states (e.g., false beliefs) compared to mental states that do not require representation about mental states (e.g., true beliefs), (3) the ToM network should show a significantly stronger response to representations about mental states (false beliefs) than to representations about physical states (e.g., false signs), (4) the ToM network should not differentiate between non-mental stories, regardless of whether they require representational abilities or not. Based on these criteria, two candidate brain regions were identified that are supposed to underlie the ToM network: the dorsal part of medial prefrontal cortex (DMPFC) and the temporo-parietal junction (TPJ). While neuroscientists agree that both brain regions are involved in belief reasoning in general, there is still debate about which of the two brain regions is specifically associated with ToM (for reviews on neuroimaging evidence on false belief understanding see Amodio & Frith, 2006; Frith & Frith, 2006; Frith & Frith, 2003; Gallagher & Frith, 2003; Saxe, 2006; Saxe & Baron-Cohen, 2006; Saxe et al., 2004).

Researchers supporting the DMPFC as being necessarily and specifically associated with ToM presented stories and cartoons which required a mixture of mental state inferences (e.g., second-order false and true belief reasoning; lack of knowledge; Fletcher et al., 1995; Gallagher et al., 2000). For example, in a PET study, Fletcher et al. (1995) presented stories that described a character who acts based on another character's true or false belief. The belief stories were contrasted with physical stories, which described a character's causal actions. As a baseline, vignettes of unlinked sentences were presented. Fletcher et al. (1995) observed that the DMPFC and the TPJ were involved in processing ToM stories compared to physical stories. In addition, while the authors did not observe DMPFC activity for physical stories compared to unlinked sentences, the TPJ was active for this contrast. Based on these findings, the authors argue for the DMPFC as subserving ToM because it was specifically active for the ToM stories. They further argued that the TPJ seems to be involved in more basic informational processes. These findings attained additional support by an fMRI study that presented both verbal and non-verbal material (Gallagher et al., 2000). With respect to the verbal material, the authors presented the same stories as in the Fletcher et al. (1995) study. With respect to the nonverbal material, the authors presented cartoons that depicted a mixture of false beliefs and lack of knowledge. In the non-ToM cartoons, no inferences on false beliefs or lack of knowledge were required. In the baseline condition, subjects were required to decode scrambled pictures. The results were similar to the Fletcher et al. (1995) study. The DMPFC and the TPJ were found to be involved in both the ToM stories and the ToM cartoons, compared to the non-ToM trials. In addition, while there was no DMPFC activity for physical trials compared to unlinked trials, the TPJ was active for this contrast.

Researchers who argue for a special role of the TPJ instead of the DMPFC in false belief understanding point out that, in addition to the ToM stimuli, the non-ToM material could have invited participants to engage on mental state reasoning because it depicts acting characters (Saxe & Kanwisher, 2003). The authors, therefore, point out that the TPJ activity observed in the 'non-ToM' stories over the baseline trials could show that the TPJ is also involved in the ToM network. Further, it can be argued that the ToM stories were not controlled for first-order false belief reasoning because they required participants to engage in a mixture of mental state inferences (e.g., second-order false and true belief reasoning, lack of knowledge). When interpreting the results on a more conservative level, they show that both the TPJ and the DMPFC are involved in belief reasoning in general. However, whether there is a specific role for both or either brain region with respect to first-order false belief remains to be explored.

Subsequent studies addressed the methodological shortcomings of the earlier studies and developed better-controlled material (Aichhorn et al., 2008f; Perner et al., 2006; Saxe & Kanwisher, 2003; Saxe & Powell, 2006; Saxe, Schulz, & Jiang, 2006; Saxe & Wexler, 2005; Sommer et al., 2007). For example, researchers who argue for a special role of the TPJ in false belief understanding contrasted first-order false belief stories with false photograph stories (Aichhorn et al., 2008e; Perner et al., 2006; Saxe & Kanwisher, 2003; Saxe & Powell, 2006; Saxe et al., 2006; Saxe & Wexler, 2005). While false belief stories are supposed to require participants to engage in representational activity about mental states, false photograph stories are supposed to be based on representations about physical states. This contrast could help clarify criterion 3 with respect to the ToM network: the ToM network should show a significantly stronger response to representations about mental states than to representations about physical states. For the false belief versus false photograph contrast the authors reported results both based on a whole brain analysis and on a functional region-of-interest analysis (fROI). Within the fROI analysis, to confirm a special role of the TPJ in false belief understanding, the authors analyzed several other contrasts in addition to the false belief versus false photograph contrast. They did not, however, report results for these fROI contrasts on a whole brain level. Contrasts that are based on fROI results, however, have to be confirmed on a whole brain level of analysis to be more reliable (Friston, Rotshtein, Geng, Sterzer,

& Henson, 2006; Stone & Gerrans, 2006). Therefore, the fROI findings, which should support a special role of the TPJ in false belief understanding, can be questioned. With respect to the whole brain results for the contrast false belief versus false photograph, Saxe and colleagues (Saxe & Kanwisher, 2003; Saxe & Powell, 2006; Saxe et al., 2006; Saxe & Wexler, 2005), and Perner and colleagues (Aichhorn et al., 2008d; Perner et al., 2006) observed that both the DMPFC and the TPJ were found to be involved in false belief over false photograph trials. Although the assumption of a special role of the TPJ instead of the DMPFC has to be questioned, the whole brain results, however, could support criterion 3 with respect to the DMPFC and the TPJ, since both brain regions show a significantly stronger response to representations about mental states than to representations about physical states.

Recent empirical evidence from developmental psychology, however, shows that the false photograph task does not require a representational understanding (Perner & Leekam, 2008) because, unlike the false belief task, the false photo task does not require the computation of true / false perspective differences in relation to the same time point. That is because the physical photo content is related to something that has been true in the past. Therefore, the physical photo content does not have to be processed independent of reality cues. The false sign task is supposed to better control for a representational understanding because the physical sign content is manipulated to be false with respect to reality. Therefore, along with the false belief task, the false sign task is argued to require computing true / false perspective differences in relation to the same time point. In two fMRI studies, Perner and colleagues (Aichhorn et al., 2008c; Perner et al., 2006) presented both the false photo and false sign condition as a control condition for the false belief task. In the false belief task Perner and colleagues presented verbal vignettes that described a present situation that was manipulated to be different from a character's belief in relation to the same time point. Parallel to the false belief task, in the false sign task the authors presented verbal vignettes that also described a present situation that was manipulated to be different from the real situation in relation to the same time point. Unfortunately, Perner and colleagues (Aichhorn et al., 2008b; Perner et al., 2006) only reported false belief over false sign results based on an fROI analysis. Functional ROI results suggest a specific role of the TPJ for ToM with respect to criterion three. As mentioned before, however, fROI results lack a strong empirical basis and have to be confirmed by a whole brain analysis. Therefore, it is still unclear, on a whole brain level, whether the DMPFC and the TPJ show significantly stronger responses to representations about mental states (false beliefs) than to representations about physical states (e.g., false signs). Fortunately, Perner et al. (2006) report results, based on a whole brain analysis, that tackle criterion 4: the ToM network should not differentiate between non-mental stories regardless of whether they require representational abilities or not. For false sign stories over physical control stories that did not require a representational understanding, the DMPFC was not involved. Within the TPJ, the authors found a hemispheric dissociation. While the right TPJ (RTPJ) as well as the DMPFC was not associated with a representational understanding of physical states, the left TPJ (LTPJ) was. These results exclude a role for the DMPFC and the RTPJ for a representational understanding of physical states.

In a recent fMRI study, our group explored the ToM network with respect to true and false belief reasoning on a whole brain analysis (Sommer et al., 2007). In parallel tasks, picture stories were presented that required subjects to engage in either true or false belief reasoning. The picture stories were modified from the original "Sally-Anne-Scenario" that was developed to test false belief understanding (Baron-Cohen et al., 1985). The dorsal part of the anterior cingulate cortex (dACC) that can be seen as the posterior region of the medial frontal cortex (prMFC) and the RTPJ showed an activity increase for the false belief over true belief contrast. By contrast, both brain regions did not responded significantly to the conjunction of true and false beliefs. With respect to the ToM network, these results could help clarify criterion 1 (the ToM network should respond to belief reasoning in general, both true and false beliefs) and criterion 2 (the ToM network should show significantly stronger responses to mental states that require representation about mental states (e.g., false beliefs) compared to mental states that do not require representation about mental states (e.g., true beliefs)). With respect to criterion 1, the conjunction results show that neither within the DMPFC nor within the TPJ is there one single brain region that responds both to false beliefs and true beliefs. In regard to criterion 2, both the DMPFC and the RTPJ are associated with representations about mental states compared to mental states that do not require representation about mental states.

With respect to the criteria defining the ToM network, results support an important role for the DMPFC and the RTPJ in false belief reasoning. Both brain regions respond significantly stronger to false than to true beliefs (criterion 2). Further, both brain regions do not differentiate between non-mental stories, regardless of whether they require representational abilities or not (criterion 4: false sign versus photo). Regarding the generality criteria, there is no single brain region within the DMPFC and the TPJ that processes both true and false beliefs (criterion 1). Criterion 1, however, needs to be further explored by contrasting both true and false belief reasoning with a non-mental control condition. In addition, whether the DMPFC and the RTPJ have a specific role in computing false beliefs over false signs remains to be explored by a whole brain analysis (criterion 3).

The criteria defining the ToM network are based on domain-specific considerations. Domain-general Theory of Mind accounts, however, challenge the specificity criterion of the ToM network. Developmental and functional findings on domain-general processes show that false belief reasoning is closely related to low-level processes such as attention or inhibition, and with more high-level processes such as language or episodic memory (for a review on developmental evidence see Sodian & Thoermer, 2006; for reviews on functional evidence see Buckner & Carroll, 2007; Corbetta, Patel, & Shulman, 2008; Hassabis & Maguire, 2007; Lieberman, 2007; Mitchell, 2006; Perner & Aichhorn, 2008; Stone & Gerrans, 2006).

In sum, domain-specific ToM accounts reveal an important role of the DMPFC and the RTPJ in false belief reasoning. Domain-general accounts, however, suggest that although the DMPFC and the RTPJ are important brain regions underlying false belief understanding, these regions may not be exclusively related to Theory of Mind. Instead, domain-general ToM accounts suggest that the DMPFC and the RTPJ are associated with more basic information processes. Nevertheless, the DMPFC and the RTPJ have turned out to be important candidate regions subserving false belief understanding.

1.2.2 Intention attribution

Although there is no neuroimaging study on intention-based emotion attribution, several neuroimaging studies have been conducted on inferring intentions from physical stimuli such as nonverbal comic strips (Brunet et al., 2000; Walter et al., 2004) or animated geometrical shapes (Castelli et al., 2002; Gobbini et al., 2007; Martin & Weisberg, 2003; Schultz, 2005; Tavares et al., 2008). The material was adopted from developmental research on intention attribution in normally developing children (Montgomery & Montgomery, 1999) and autistic children (Abell, Happe, & Frith, 2000; Baron-Cohen, Leslie, & Frith, 1986)

Regarding the DMPFC and the RTPJ as candidate regions within the ToM network, the majority of studies found that inferring intentions from physical cues recruits the DMPFC (nonverbal comic strips: Brunet et al., 2000; Walter et al., 2004; animated geometrical shapes: Castelli, Happe, Frith, & Frith, 2000; Gobbini et al., 2007; Schultz et al., 2003; Tavares et al., 2008; Vanderwal, Hunyadi, Grupe, Connors, & Schultz, 2008). The majority of studies, however, did not observe RTPJ recruitment. Rather than the RTPJ, these studies found that inferring intentions from physical cues was associated with large activation patterns in temporal regions, including the superior, middle, and inferior temporal cortex, the fusiform gyrus, and the temporal poles. These results suggest that intention attribution compared to false belief reasoning is associated with common activity in the DMPFC. In contrast, RTPJ activity seems to be associated with false belief reasoning rather than with intention attribution.

Three studies, however, found RTPJ activity associated with intention attribution (nonverbal comic strips: Walter et al., 2004; animated geometrical shapes: Martin & Weisberg, 2003; Schultz et al., 2003). This RTPJ activity, however, could be due to methodological shortcomings. The studies used block designs, which also included response trials such as logical reasoning. Therefore, the RTPJ activity could also be an effect of other cognitive processes rather than an effect of intention attribution. In addition, Walter et al. (2004) contrasted an intention attribution condition involving characters with a physical control condition without characters. Therefore, RTPJ activity could also be caused by the involvement of characters rather than by intention attribution.

These considerations on methodological limitations, probably being due to RTPJ activity, are supported by two studies on intention attribution which either used a physical control condition involving characters (Brunet et al., 2000) or used an event-related approach (Tavares et al., 2008). In a PET study, Brunet et al. (2000) presented nonverbal comic strips adopted from a developmental study on intention attribution in autistic children (Baron-Cohen et al., 1986). In the intention attribution condition, an acting character was depicted. The target picture was presented along with two distracter pictures, which did not match the character's intention. In addition to the intention condition, the authors presented two control conditions, which depicted physical causality. To control for the involvement of characters, one physical causality condition involved a character. The second physical causality condition involved no character. Attribution of intention compared to physical causality involving a character was associated with activity in the DMPFC, the lateral prefrontal cortex and the temporal poles. RTPJ activity was not observed in this contrast. Physical causality with characters compared to physical causalities without character activated the left TPJ, the temporal pole, the fusiform gyrus, and temporal brain regions. These results support the view that intention attribution is rather associated with prefrontal brain regions than with posterior brain regions, including the TPJ.

A recent fMRI study on intention attribution used parallel material in an event-related approach (Tavares et al., 2008). The authors presented animations of two geometrical shapes and included obstacles to motion. In order to broadly sample different interpersonal situations, they presented three categories of animations (friendly, antagonistic, indifferent). Following the animation probe, statements were presented which described the contents of the animation. The animation epoch and the response epoch were separately analysed. In the intention attribution condition participants were instructed to attend to the social behaviour that could underlie the motion of the geometrical shapes. In the control condition participants had to attend to spatial, non-mental, properties with respect to the moving characters. In the response epoch of the intention attribution condition, participants had to judge, on a true/false dimension, if the statement could appropriately describe the behaviour in the animation. In the response epoch of the control condition participants had to decide on statements regarding these physical properties. Whole brain analysis results showed that in the animation epoch the DMPFC was the only brain region which responded significantly to attention on intention attribution compared to attention on physical properties. In the response epoch, together with the parahippocampal cortex, the DMPFC also responded significantly to intention attribution compared to the physical control condition. These results also support the assumption that the DMPFC is involved in intention attribution.

Another recent fMRI study compared belief reasoning and intention attribution in the same adult sample (Gobbini et al., 2007). In the belief task the authors used verbal stories adopted from Fletcher et al. (1995) and nonverbal cartoons adopted from Gallagher et al. (2000). In the intention condition they presented animations of geometrical shapes adopted from Castelli et al. (2000). Both the belief and the intention trials showed activity in the DMPFC. However, there was only partial overlap within the DMPFC and no overlap in the TPJ. While belief reasoning was associated with activity more in the rostral part of the medial frontal cortex, intention attribution showed activity in more posterior parts of the DMPFC. In addition, while the TPJ was recruited for belief reasoning, intention attribution showed activity in the posterior superior temporal sulcus (pSTS) along with activity in the mirror neuron system (MNS, Iacoboni, 2008; Iacoboni & Dapretto, 2006). The pSTS and the MNS are supposed to be involved in the action perception, with the MNS having a special role in understanding intentional motor activity. Based on their findings, the authors suggest that two nearby regions, the TPJ and the pSTS, play dissociable roles in the understanding of different mental states such as beliefs or intentions. They suggest that whereas the TPJ may play a role in the processing of mental states, which cannot be inferred by physical properties, the pSTS may play a role in the representation of perceived actions, and along with the mirror neuron system, the representation of intentions that are inferred from those physical actions.

In sum, neuroimaging findings on intention attribution from physical cues such as nonverbal comic strips and animated geometrical shapes suggest that both false belief reasoning and intention attribution are associated with only partially overlapping brain regions in the DMPFC. While false belief reasoning seems to be associated more with rostral parts of the medial prefrontal cortex, intention attribution seems to rely on activity in more posterior parts of the DMPFC (Fig. 1.1). In contrast to the DMPFC activity being involved in both false belief and intention understanding, the TPJ seems to be recruited during false belief reasoning rather than intention attribution. Intention attribution seems to rely more on activity in the pSTS and the MNS. These results suggest that the medial prefrontal cortex rather than the TPJ plays an important role not only in false belief reasoning but also in intention attribution. Moreover, these results may show that false belief reasoning and intention attribution are associated with both overlapping and distinct networks. Functional results therefore suggest that false belief understanding and intention attribution from physical cues rely on both common and distinct information processes.

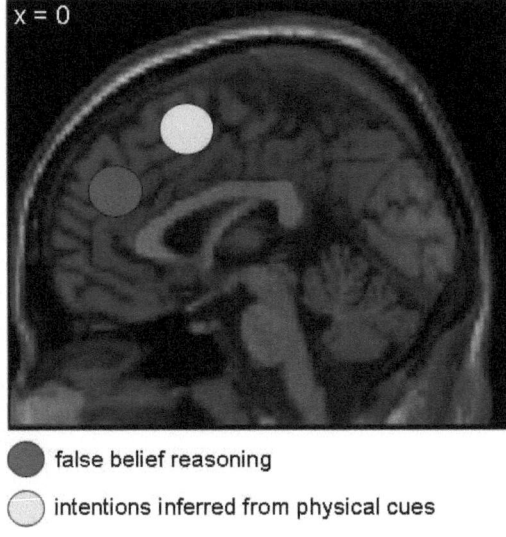

Fig. 1.1: Involvement of the medial prefrontal cortex in ToM. More rostral parts of the medial prefrontal cortex (MPFC) are associated with false belief reasoning (red), more posterior parts of the MPFC are associated with the understanding of intentions inferred from physical cues (yellow).

1.2.3 Emotion attribution

In addition to studies that have explored the neural network associated with intention attribution inferred from physical cues, there are several studies that have explored emotion attribution inferred from physical cues such as affective eye gazes (Baron-Cohen et al., 1999; Wicker et al., 2003), affective faces (Schulte-Ruther et al., 2007) and pictures (Ochsner et al., 2004), affective point-light walkers (Heberlein & Saxe, 2005), and affective verbal vignettes (Hynes et al., 2006; Ruby & Decety, 2004). Among those studies there are, however, only two studies that compared, on the level of a whole brain analysis, emotion attribution with a non-mental control condition in healthy adults (Ochsner et al., 2004; Wicker et al., 2003). The other studies cited above either reported results based on a region-of-interest analysis rather than on a whole brain analysis (Hynes et al., 2006), or reported results for emotion attribution alone without directly comparing emotion attribution with the non-mental control condition (Baron-Cohen et al., 1999), or compared self versus other judgements in emotion attribution without reporting results for attributing emotions to others compared to a non-mental control condition (Ruby & Decety, 2004; Schulte-Ruther et al., 2007), or compared emotion attribution with judgements about personality traits (Heberlein & Saxe,

2005). The personality traits condition contained social-moral emotions such as trustworthiness and friendliness. Therefore, there is only little functional evidence with respect to the neural correlates associated with emotion attribution within the Theory of Mind research field (Olsson & Ochsner, 2008).

In a PET study, Wicker et al. (2003) compared emotions inferred from affective eye gaze with attentional judgements inferred from neutral eye gaze. Emotion attribution was associated with activity in the dorsal and ventral part of the medial prefrontal cortex, the bilateral temporal cortex, including the temporal poles, and the posterior cingulate / precuneus. These results, however, have to be interpreted with caution because emotion attribution confounds with the emotional material, since in the control condition neutral rather than emotional faces were presented. An fMRI study conducted by Ochsner et al. (2004) was controlled for these confounding effects. They compared emotion attribution inferred from positive, negative and neutral pictures with nonmental judgements inferred from the same set of stimuli. Emotion attribution was found to be associated with activity in the DMPFC, the bilateral middle temporal cortex, the precuneus, the middle occipital cortex, and the parahippocampal gyrus.

In sum, with respect to the neural network associated with false belief reasoning, emotion attribution inferred from physical cues is particularly associated with activity in the DMPFC. Instead of TPJ activity, emotion attribution seems to be more associated with activity in the temporal cortex. As with intention attribution and false belief understanding, the medial prefrontal cortex rather than the TPJ may play an important role in emotion attribution inferred from physical cues. As with intention attribution, emotions inferred from physical cues seem to be associated more with activity in temporal brain regions. These results suggest that false belief understanding, intention attribution, and inferring emotions from physical cues are associated with both overlapping and distinct networks. While intention and emotion attribution seem to rely on similar networks, there seems to be only an overlap with false belief understanding in the DMPFC. These results suggest that the DMPFC plays an important role in mental state attribution in general. Moreover, these results may show that while intention and emotion attribution are associated with similar information processes, false belief understanding may require, at least in part, distinct information processes.

1.3 Summary and research question

Although there are several neuroimaging studies on intention and emotion attribution inferred from physical cues, this is the first study which explores the neural network associated with emotion attribution based on other mental states such as intentions. Therefore, it is still an open question whether intention-based emotion attribution and belief reasoning are associated with common or distinct neural networks. Experiment one of this thesis investigates emotion attribution based on intention-outcome-relations.

Developmental findings suggest distinct neural networks because the ability for emotion attribution based on intention-outcome-relations shortly precedes the ability for false belief understanding. Specifically, with respect to mental state understanding, there seems to be a change from taking an objective stance in 2½- to 4-year-olds to a subjective stance in 4- to 5-year-olds. Functional findings on false belief reasoning revealed an important role for the dorsal medial prefrontal cortex (DMPFC) and the temporo-parietal junction (TPJ), particularly the right TPJ (RTPJ). Neuroimaging studies on intention and emotion attribution inferred from physical cues observed both distinct and common neural networks in relation to false belief understanding. Distinct activity was found in more posterior brain regions. The TPJ was observed to be more associated with false belief understanding, while temporal brain regions were found to be more associated with intention and emotion attribution. Common activity was found in frontal brain regions, particularly the DMPFC. Based on the developmental and functional findings, it is hypothesized that intention-based emotion attribution would be associated with both distinct and common neural networks with respect to false belief understanding. It is predicted that the medial prefrontal cortex, particularly the DMPFC would be associated with intention-based emotion. Furthermore, it is predicted that more posterior brain regions, particularly the TPJ, would be less associated with intention-based emotion attribution.

To explore emotion attribution based on intention-outcome-relations, nonverbal stories with verbal vignettes were presented. The material was adopted from developmental studies on intention-based emotion attribution. In the emotion attribution conditions, a protagonist's intention either matched (intention fulfilled) or mismatched the outcome of the intended action (intention unfulfilled). In addition to the emotion attribution condition, a paralleled non-mental control condition was used.

2. METHODS

STUDY I
EMOTIONS INFERRED FROM INTENTION-OUTCOME-RELATIONS

2.1 Participants

Fourteen right-handed male subjects (age range = 22-45 years, M = 31.64 years, SD = 6.80 years) with no neurological or psychiatric history participated in the study. All participants gave informed consent according to the guidelines of the local Ethic Committee.

2.2 Task and material

Intention-based emotion attribution was explored by a modified, fMRI compatible version adopted from the developmental study of Yuill et al. (1996). Cartoons that were described by verbal vignettes were presented. The nonverbal pictures depicted three children playing, a protagonist and two recipients (Figs. 2.1 and 2.2). Eight story contexts were used: children playing with a ball, a teddy, a balloon, a toy airplane, a toy duck, a toy car, badminton, or hockey. The nonverbal material was held equivalent across the study conditions, which only differed in their verbal vignettes. Two emotion attribution conditions were realized which varied on the factor 'intention-outcome-relation' (Fig. 2.1). The factor 'intention-outcome-relation' varied on whether the protagonist's intention matched (fulfilled intention) or mismatched the outcome situation (unfulfilled intention). Moreover, a non-mental control condition was realized that solely described physical processes (Fig. 2.2).

In both emotion attribution conditions the verbal vignette in the first story picture described the protagonist's intention (e.g., 'Max wants to throw the ball to Lena'; 'Anna wants to roll the duck to Tim'). Emotion attribution conditions differed in the second story picture which presented the outcome of the intended action (fulfilled intention: e.g., 'Max throws the ball to Lena; unfulfilled intention: e.g., 'Anna rolls the duck to Marie'). In the third picture the protagonist was depicted and the participants were instructed to reason about the protagonist's emotion dependent on its prior intention and on the outcome of the intended action ('How does...feel?'). To separate reasoning about the actor's emotion from giving a motor response, participants were instructed not to respond before the response stimulus was presented. The response stimulus depicted three smileys (neutral, positive, negative). Responses were given by pressing a button.

In the reality condition verbal vignettes in the first two pictures described the scene (e.g., picture 1: 'The kids are playing with the puck'; picture 2: 'Max has the puck'). In the third picture participants were instructed to reason about the toy the kids were playing with ('What is...playing with?'). In the fourth picture stimulus the target toy was presented along with two distracter toys. Here, participants were instructed to respond to the target toy by pressing a button.

For each condition 34 trials were presented. In order to reduce response predictability in the emotion attribution conditions, 15 % control trials were presented along with the experimental trials. In these control trials participants had to reason about the emotional state of one of the recipients instead of reasoning about the protagonist's emotional state. These trials were not included in the analysis. Stimulus complexity was held equivalent across conditions. The protagonist's and the recipients' gender was counterbalanced, as well as the protagonist's presentation side on the screen (left/right). All children were presented without a facial expression in order not to trigger specific emotion attribution processes by the visual input. In the response trials the presentation order of the smileys and of the toys was counterbalanced.

In order to obtain more specific emotion attribution responses, a rating task was conducted following the scanning session (Appendix B). In the rating task the same cartoon-stories were presented as in the experimental task and the same emotion attribution conditions were used. Five trials were presented in each emotion attribution condition. Participants were instructed to rate the actor's emotion on six emotion dimensions (neutral, happiness, sadness, embarrassment, surprise, anger). Each dimension varied on a five-point Likert scale ranging from 1 (not at all) to 5 (very strong). One rating data set was excluded from the analysis because of too many missing data. Therefore, thirteen data sets were included in the analysis of the rating data.

2.3 Experimental procedure

Prior to the experimental task participants attended a training session to become familiar with the stimulus material. Following the fMRI session, the rating task was conducted. During the fMRI session stimuli were back-projected onto a screen. Foam padding restricted head motion. Conditions were randomly presented across the scanning session. Within each trial stimuli were presented in a fixed order: the story stimuli (pictures 1 and 2) were presented for 2.5 seconds each. The emotion attribution stimulus and the reality processing stimulus (picture 3) were presented for 6 seconds each. The response stimulus (picture 4) was presented for 2 seconds. Time varying fixation periods were presented before each trial (2-4 sec) and before the third picture (1-3 sec). Fixation periods were included to measure an inter-stimulus baseline and to properly model the hemodynamic response function associated with emotion attribution. Presentation software was used for stimulus presentation and for response recording (Neurobehavioral Systems Inc., Albany, CA). Responses were recorded by using three buttons of a five-button fMRI compatible response pad (LUMItouch, Photon Control Inc., Burnaby, Canada).

Study I – Methods

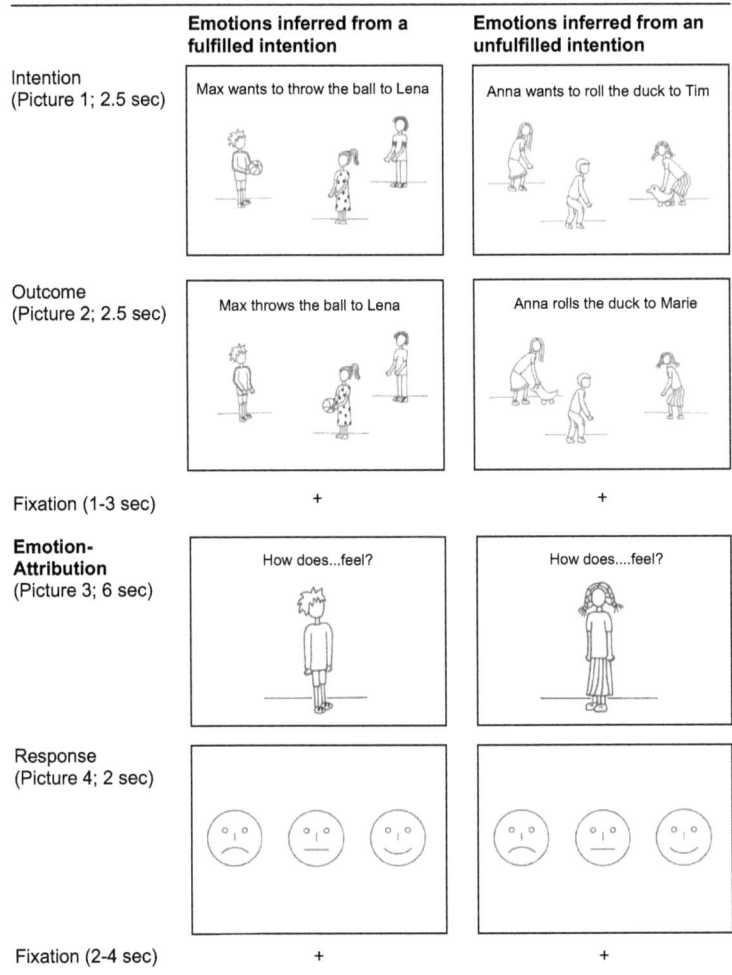

Fig. 2.1: Example of emotion attribution based on a fulfilled intention (left) and an unfulfilled intention (right). Pictures were consecutively presented with intermediate fixation periods varying in time intervals. Functional analysis focused on the emotion attribution stimuli (picture 3).

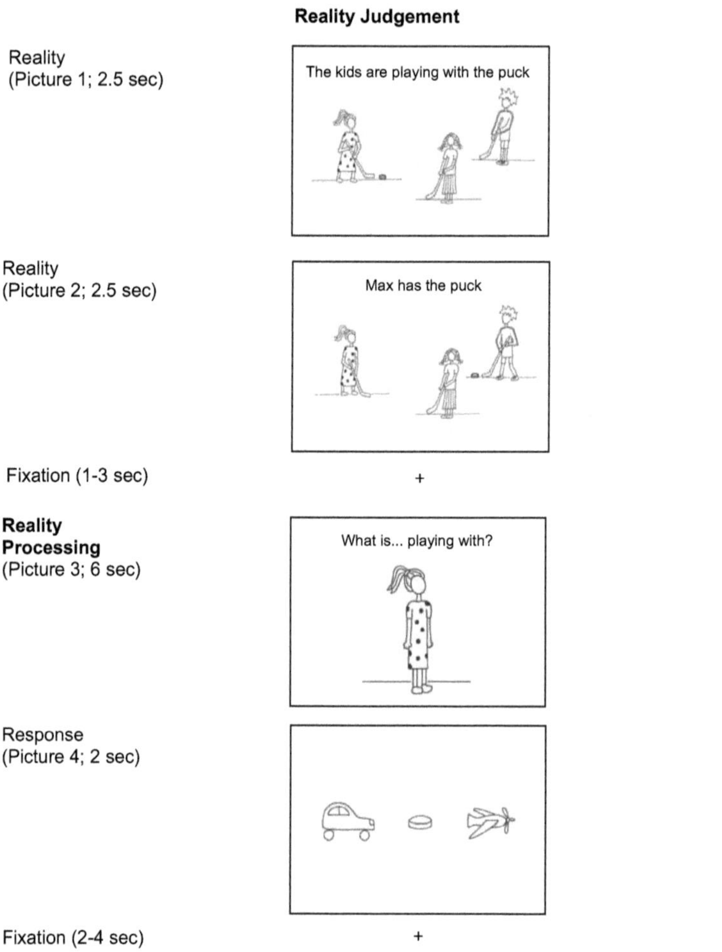

Study I – Methods

Reality Judgement

Reality
(Picture 1; 2.5 sec)

> The kids are playing with the puck

Reality
(Picture 2; 2.5 sec)

> Max has the puck

Fixation (1-3 sec)

+

Reality Processing
(Picture 3; 6 sec)

> What is... playing with?

Response
(Picture 4; 2 sec)

Fixation (2-4 sec)

+

Fig. 2.2: Example of a reality judgement trial. Pictures were consecutively presented with intermediate fixation periods varying in time intervals. Functional analysis focused on the reality processing stimuli (picture 3).

2.4 Statistical analysis of the behavioural data

The statistical analysis of the behavioural data was conducted with SPSS 15. In the reality condition response accuracy (in percentage) was analysed. With respect to the emotion attribution responses obtained during the scanning session, for every emotion dimension (neutral, positive, negative) the mean percentage of emotion responses out of its total amount was calculated. In the rating task for every emotion dimension (neutral, happiness, sadness, embarrassment, surprise, anger) a mean rating score ranging from 1 (not at all) to 5 (very strong) was computed. For every emotion dimension statistical comparisons were done for the two experimental conditions (match: intention fulfilled; mismatch: intention unfulfilled) by conducting paired t-tests with Greenhouse-Geisser alpha-correction. T-tests were two-tailed and a value of $p \leq .05$ was used to determine statistical significance.

2.5 Imaging and image preprocessing

Scanning was performed in an interleaved fashion on a 1.5 Tesla fMRI scanner (Siemens Sonata, Erlangen, Germany). The functional images sensitive to blood oxygenation level dependent (BOLD) contrasts were acquired by T2*-weighted echo planar images (EPI, TR = 2.82 sec, TE = 40 ms, flip angle = 90°, in plane matrix 64 x 64, FoV = 192 mm). The images consisted of 32 axial slices with 3 mm thickness and 3 x 3 mm in plane resolution. During the scanning 720 volumes were acquired. High resolution structural weighted images (TR = 1.97 sec, TE = 3.93 ms, TI = 1100 ms, voxel size 1 x 1 x 1 mm, 176 axial slices, FoV = 250 mm) were recorded from all participants. The scanning session lasted approximately 40 min.

All images were preprocessed using the SPM5 software package (http://www.fil.ion.ucl.ac.uk/spm/) and the MATLAB 7.0 software (The MathWorks Inc., Natick, MA). For each participant functional images were slice-time corrected using the middle slice as reference, realigned to the first volume by rigid body transformation to correct for participants' motion, normalised to the Montreal Neurological Institute (MNI) reference brain (Collins, Neelin, Peters, & Evans, 1994), and spatially smoothed by a Gaussian kernel with a full-width half-maximum of 8mm.

2.6 Statistical analysis of the images

All statistical first and second-level analysis were conducted with the SPM5 software package and were based on the entire brain. The analysis focused on amplitude changes in the hemodynamic response function (HRF) associated with emotion attribution and reality judgement (picture 3). Fixation periods served to measure an inter-stimulus baseline and to analyse the hemodynamic response function associated with emotion attribution and reality judgement.

In the first-level analysis a fixed effects analysis was computed for each participant based on the general linear model (GLM). The stimuli were modelled by boxcars of 5 seconds, which were then convolved with the HRF, along with its time and dispersion derivatives to account for any temporal and spatial shifts in the response of the stimuli (Friston et al., 1998). Also included were six covariates to capture residual movement-related artefacts and a single covariate representing the mean (constant) over scans. The data were high-pass filtered with a frequency cutoff at 128 seconds. Statistical parametric maps (SPMs) were generated for each subject by t-statistics derived from contrasts utilizing the HRF (Friston et al., 2002). The derivates from the statistical model were not included in the contrasts.

These contrasts of interest were computed on the individual analysis level:

Contrast 1: emotion attribution versus reality judgement ('Fulfilled Intention' + 'Unfulfilled Intention' versus 'Non-Ment')

Contrast 2: Emotions inferred from unfulfilled intentions versus reality judgement ('Unfulfilled Intention' versus 'Non-Ment')

Contrast 3: Emotions inferred from fulfilled intentions versus reality judgement ('Fulfilled Intention' versus 'Non-Ment')

Contrast 4: Emotions inferred from unfulfilled versus fulfilled intentions ('Unfulfilled Intention' versus 'Fulfilled Intention')

These single-subject first-level contrast images from the weighted beta-images were introduced into second-level random-effects analysis to allow for population inference. For each contrast one-sample t-tests were conducted. All fMRI results reported here are based on voxel statistics computed with SPM for the entire brain. The resulting set of significant voxel values for each contrast constituted an SPM map. The maps were thresholded at $T = 3.79$ ($p \leq .001$ uncorrected), overlaid on the MNI template, and labelled by using the MNI coordinates. For graphical purposes in those brain regions showing significant effects mean cluster values (parameter estimates) were extracted by using the SPM5 software.

3. RESULTS

STUDY I
EMOTIONS INFERRED FROM INTENTION-OUTCOME-RELATIONS

3.1 Behavioural findings

The emotion attribution results obtained during the fMRI session are shown in Table 3.1 and Figure 3.1. Mean hitrate for the reality judgement was 98 % (SD = 4 %). Regarding emotion attribution results, significantly more positive emotions were attributed based on a fulfilled relative to an unfulfilled intention ($t(13)$ = 8.14, $p \leq .001$). In contrast, more neutral and negative emotions were attributed based on an unfulfilled compared to a fulfilled intention ($t(13)$ = 3.38, $p \leq .01$).

Table 3.1: Mean emotion attribution scores of the fMRI session for the intention fulfilled and intention unfulfilled emotion attribution condition.

Emotion[a]	Fulfilled Intention		Unfulfilled Intention	
	M	(SD)	M	(SD)
Neutral	9	(13)	27	(28)
Positive	84	(19)	16	(20)
Negative	7	(8)	57	(33)

Notes: M, mean; SD, standard deviation.
[a] Percentage of neutral, positive, and negative responses out of the total amount of emotion responses

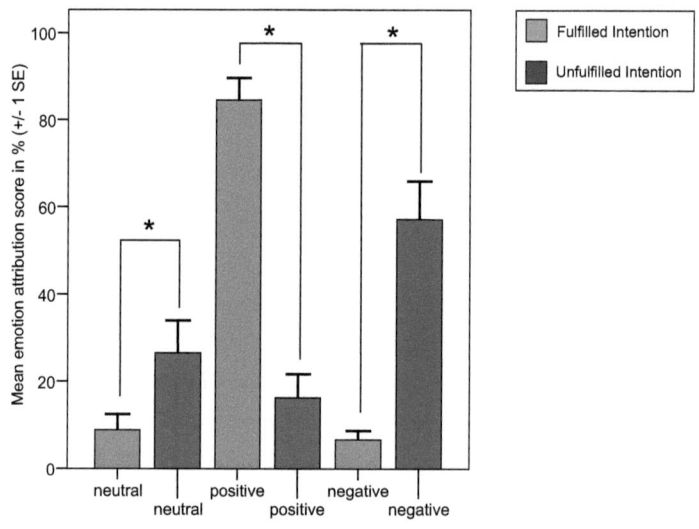

Fig. 3.1: Main effect of the factor intention-outcome-relation. Results were obtained during the fMRI session. Mean emotion attribution scores (+/-1 SE) in the intention fulfilled (light grey) compared to the intention unfulfilled emotion attribution condition (dark grey).

More specific emotion attribution results were obtained during the rating task that followed the fMRI session (Tab. 3.2, Fig. 3.2). The rating results confirmed the emotion attribution results obtained in the fMRI session. On a rating scale ranging from 1 (not at all) to 5 (very strong), significantly more happiness was attributed based on a fulfilled compared to an unfulfilled intention ($t(12) = 8.56$, $p \leq .001$). In contrast, significantly more sadness ($t(12) = 5.70$, $p \leq .001$), surprise ($t(12) = 3.84$, $P \leq .01$), embarrassment ($t(12) = 6.65$, $p \leq .001$), and anger ($t(12) = 5.12$, $p \leq .001$) were attributed based on an unfulfilled compared to a fulfilled intention. For the neutral dimension no significant difference between emotion attribution conditions was observed ($t(12) = 0.86$, n.s.).

Table 3.2: Mean emotion attribution scores of the rating task for the intention fulfilled and intention unfulfilled emotion attribution condition.

Emotion[a]	Fulfilled Intention		Unfulfilled Intention	
	M	(SD)	M	(SD)
Neutral	1.80	(1.26)	1.51	(0.66)
Happiness	4.38	(0.72)	2.00	(1.05)
Surprise	1.41	(0.66)	2.78	(1.24)
Embarrassment	1.45	(0.70)	3.48	(1.18)
Sadness	1.06	(0.23)	2.78	(1.20)
Anger	1.06	(0.23)	2.75	(1.16)

Notes: M, mean; SD, standard deviation.
[a] Rating scores range from 1 (not at all) to 5 (very strong)

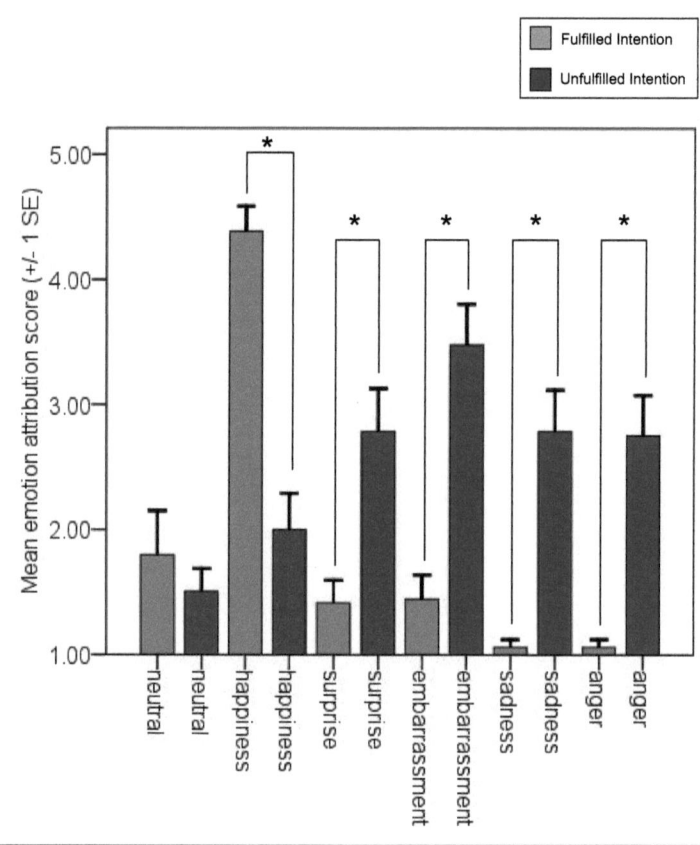

Fig. 3.2: Main effect of the factor intention-outcome-relation. Results were obtained during the rating task. Mean emotion attribution scores (+/-1 SE; 1 = not at all; 5 = very strong) in the intention fulfilled (light grey) compared to the intention unfulfilled emotion attribution condition (dark grey).

3.2 Neuroimaging findings

The fMRI analysis focused on the functional activity pattern associated with emotion attribution. FMRI results are listed in Table 3.3 and shown in Figures 3.3 to 3.6. In general, emotion attribution compared to reality judgement was associated with a signal increase in the medial pre-supplementary motor area (pre-SMA, BA6), and in the right dorsolateral prefrontal cortex (DLPFC, BA9). Further, emotions inferred from fulfilled and unfulfilled intentions compared to reality judgements were both associated with an activity increase in the medial pre-SMA (BA6, Fig. 3.3). Moreover, emotions inferred from unfulfilled intentions, but not fulfilled intentions, compared to reality judgements, were associated with a signal increase in the dorso- and ventrolateral prefrontal cortex (DLPFC, BA9, Fig. 3.4; VLPFC, BA 47, Fig. 3.5). Besides activity increases in response to emotion attribution, emotion attribution was associated with a linear signal decrease in the orbital part of the paracingulate cortex (BA 32, Fig. 3.6). Specifically, emotion attribution based on unfulfilled intentions showed a significantly stronger signal decrease compared to emotion attribution based on fulfilled intentions. Further, reality judgements were associated with a significant activity increase compared to both emotion attribution conditions.

Table 3.3: Brain regions showing significant functional signal changes associated with emotion attribution.

Brain region	BA	Cluster Size[a]	t-value (df = 13)[b]	x,y,z (mm)[c]
Emotion Attribution vs Reality				
Pre-supplementary motor area	6	360	7.11[d]	-6, 6, 66
Right dorsolateral prefrontal cortex	9	145	5.33[d]	46, 16, 34
Fulfilled Intention vs Reality				
Pre-supplementary motor area	6	93	6.95[e]	-8, 2, 64
Unfulfilled Intention vs Reality				
Pre-supplementary motor area	6	215	6.35[d]	-8, 8, 64
Left ventrolateral prefrontal cortex	47	104	5.80[e]	-32, 24, -8
Right dorsolateral prefrontal cortex	9	140	5.45[d]	44, 12, 34
Fulfilled Intention vs Unfulfilled Intention				
Orbital paracingulate cortex	32	173	7.22[d]	4, 40, -8
Reality vs Unfulfilled Intention				
Orbital paracingulate cortex	32	1146	7.83[d]	6, 44, 0
Reality vs Fulfilled Intention				
Orbital paracingulate cortex	32	178	5.64[d]	8, 46, 4

Notes: BA, Brodmann's areas are approximate.
[a] Numbers of activated voxels per cluster.
[b] Peak t-value in activated cluster, df = degrees of freedom.
[c] Peak coordinate of activated cluster according to the Montreal Neurological Institute (MNI) atlas.
[d] Brain region satisfies a statistical cluster threshold of $p \leq .05$ (corrected).
[e] Brain region satisfies a statistical cluster threshold of $p \leq .01$ (corrected).

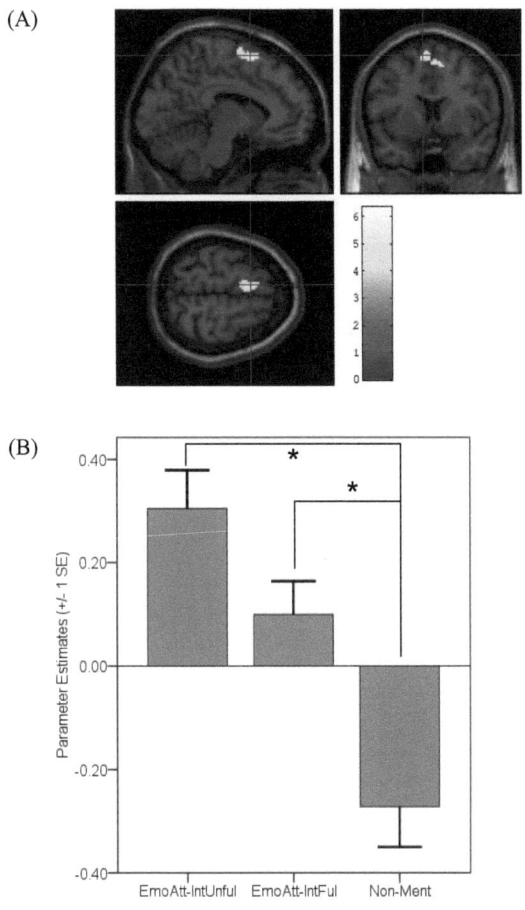

Fig. 3.3: (A) Functional changes in the amplitude of the HRF in the medial pre-SMA (BA6) associated with emotion attribution. (B) BA6 showed a significant signal increase associated with emotion attribution based on both an unfulfilled (EmoAtt-IntUnful) and fulfilled intention (EmoAtt-IntFul), compared to reality judgement (Non-Ment). HRF, hemodynamic response function; BA, Brodmann's area.

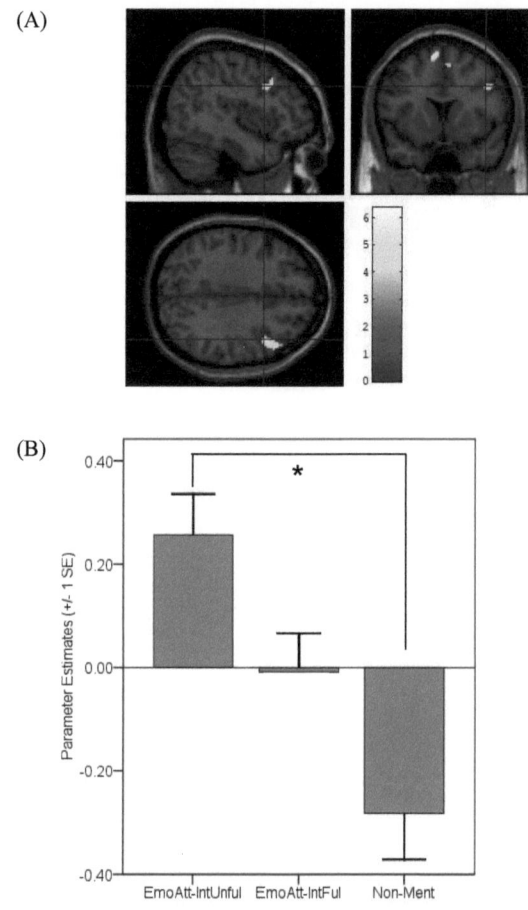

Fig. 3.4: (A) Functional changes in the amplitude of the HRF in the right dorsolateral prefrontal cortex (BA9) associated with emotion attribution. (B) BA9 showed a significant signal increase associated with emotion attribution based on an unfulfilled intention (EmoAtt-IntUnful) compared to reality judgement (Non-Ment). HRF, hemodynamic response function; BA, Brodmann's area.

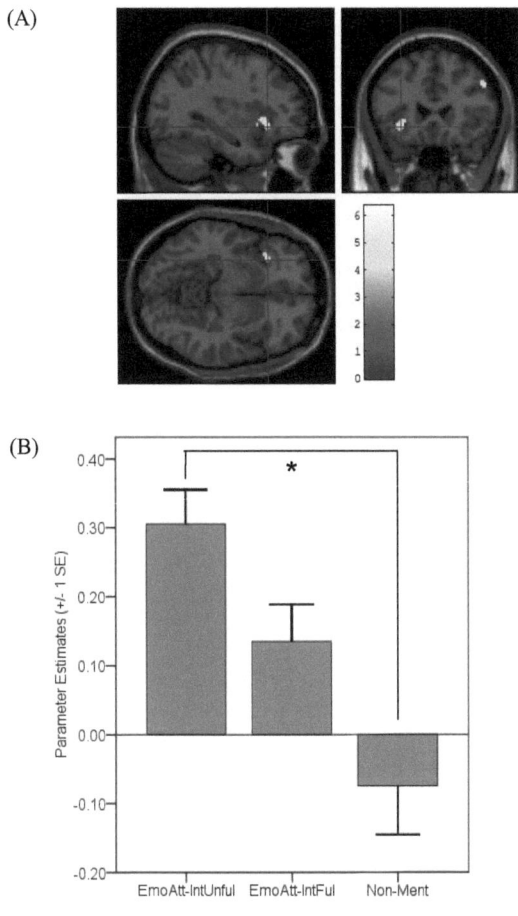

Fig. 3.5: (A) Functional changes in the amplitude of the HRF in the left ventrolateral prefrontal cortex (BA47) associated with emotion attribution. (B) BA47 showed a significant signal increase associated with emotion attribution based on a an unfulfilled intention (EmoAtt-IntUnful) compared to reality judgement (Non-Ment). HRF, hemodynamic response function; BA, Brodmann's area.

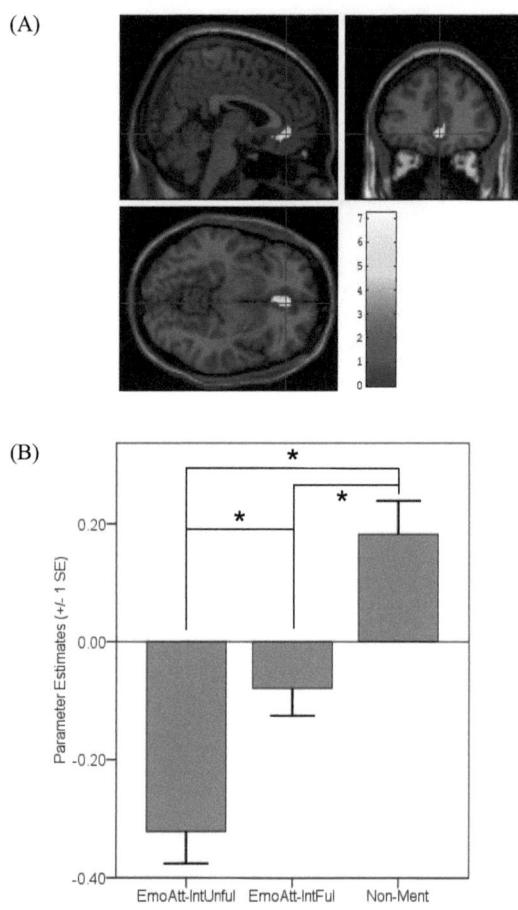

Fig. 3.6: (A) Functional changes in the amplitude of the HRF in the orbital part of the paracingulate cortex (BA32) associated with emotion attribution. (B) BA32 showed a significant signal decrease in the intention unfulfilled condition (EmoAtt-IntUnful) compared to the intention fulfilled condition (EmoAtt-IntFul) Further, reality judgements (Non-Ment) were associated with a significant activity increase compared to both emotion attribution conditions. HRF, hemodynamic response function; BA, Brodmann's area.

4. DISCUSSION

STUDY I
EMOTIONS INFERRED FROM INTENTION-OUTCOME-RELATIONS

This thesis extends research on the neural network involved in false belief reasoning, the key Theory of Mind ability, to intention-based emotion attribution. The ability to infer another person's emotions from his or her intention is closely acquired around the ability to understand false beliefs, the key ToM ability. The first experiment explored the neural network involved in emotion attribution inferred from intention-outcome-relations. In the emotion attribution conditions a protagonist's intention either matched or mismatched the outcome of the intended action. In addition to the emotion attribution condition, a paralleled non-mental control condition was used. Chapter 4.1 discusses the behavioural findings, followed by the discussion of the functional findings (chapter 4.2) and a summary (chapter 4.3).

4.1 Behavioural findings

While emotion attribution based on a fulfilled intention was associated with more positive emotions, more negative emotions were inferred from unfulfilled intentions. These results were confirmed by a rating task that followed the fMRI session. Emotions inferred from fulfilled intentions were associated with happiness ratings; emotions inferred from unfulfilled intentions were associated with more negative emotions such as sadness, surprise, embarrassment, and anger. The results are supported by a developmental study which comprised an adult sample in addition to children samples (Lagattuta, 2005). The ability to appropriately relate intentions with outcome information is required before the development of false belief understanding. By the age of 2½ to 4 years children are able to judge a person holding a neutral intention as feeling happy when a desired goal was fulfilled and as feeling sad when the desired goal was not fulfilled (Astington; Feinfield et al., 1999; Hadwin & Perner, 1991; Lagattuta, 2005; Stein & Levine, 1989; Wellman & Banerjee, 1991; Wellman & Woolley, 1990; Yuill, 1984; Yuill et al., 1996). Therefore, in the present experiment it seems that adults' ratings are based on goal-oriented considerations (Lagattuta, 2005). The ability to infer emotions from intention-outcome relations shortly develops before the ability to understand false beliefs. It is still an open question whether emotion attribution based on intention-outcome-relations is associated with common or distinct neural networks in relation to false belief reasoning.

4.2 Neuroimaging findings

Emotion attribution based on intention-outcome-relations was observed to be confined to activity in the prefrontal cortex. While the dorsolateral prefrontal cortex (DLPFC, BA 9) and the ventrolateral prefrontal cortex (VLPFC, BA 47) responded to emotions inferred from unfulfilled intentions compared to reality, the medial prefrontal cortex (MPFC) responded to emotion attribution based on fulfilled as well as unfulfilled intentions, compared to reality. Moreover, a dissociation within the MPFC was observed along a dorsal-ventral axis. While the medial pre-supplementary motor area (pre-SMA, BA 6) showed activity increases for emotion attribution based on unfulfilled and fulfilled intentions, compared to reality, the orbital part of the paracingulate cortex (BA 32) was associated with an activity decrease for both intention conditions compared to the reality condition. What follows is the discussion of the activity increase in the pre-SMA (chapter 4.2.1), the dorsolateral and ventrolateral prefrontal cortex (chapter 4.2.2 and 4.2.3) and the discussion of the activity decrease in the orbital part of the paracingulate cortex (chapter 4.2.4).

4.2.1 Activity increase in the medial pre-SMA

Intention-based emotion attribution was found to activate the medial pre-SMA. This finding is supported by neuroimaging studies on intention attribution inferred from physical cues (Brunet et al., 2000; Gobbini et al., 2007). Brunet et al. (2000) observed that the processing of intentions inferred from physical cues was associated with activity in the DMPFC, extending into premotor regions. Further support comes from Gobbini et al. (2007), who compared belief reasoning and intention attribution in the same adult sample. While belief reasoning was associated with activity more in the rostral part of the medial prefrontal cortex, intention attribution showed activity in more posterior parts of the DMPFC, extending into premotor regions. Therefore, the present findings suggest that emotions may be inferred by the processing of intentions in relation to physical cues, such as the outcome situation, rather than by processing the actor's intention independent of physical cues. In developmental terms, participants may have inferred the actor's emotion by processing the 'intended situation' (objective stance) rather than the 'actor's intention' (subjective stance). The neuroimaging findings therefore can help clarify developmental theories by providing functional evidence that even in adulthood emotions may be inferred from intention-outcome relations, and, at least in the case of neutral intentions, based on an objective stance.

Further support for the interpretation that the activity increase in the pre-SMA may indicate that participants may have inferred the actor's emotion by matching its intention to the outcome situation comes from research on mirror neurons (for reviews on the mirror neuron system see Gallese, 2007; Iacoboni & Mazziotta, 2007; Rizzolatti & Fabbri-Destro, 2008). Mirror neurons are supposed to be located in monkey and human brain regions which have a predominately or fundamentally motor function. In humans these brain regions are assumed to be the rostral part of the inferior parietal lobule (IPL), the ventral and dorsal premotor cortex, and the posterior part of the inferior frontal gyrus (IFG), including BA 44 and BA45. Mirror neurons do not only become active when performing a motor act, but they also activate during the observation of goal-centred aspects of another's motor act. Researchers on the mirror neuron system define goal-directed behaviour in terms of intentionality. Therefore, they suppose that mirror neurons process the intentionality aspects of the motor behaviour. More specifically, mirror neurons are supposed to map the sensory representation induced by action observation onto the motor representation of that same action. Researchers who support the role of mirror neurons in intention understanding emphasize that, without mapping sensory representations onto motor representations, these sensory aspects of a motor behaviour could not be processed in terms of their intentional meaning. At best, they argue, the sensory cues would provide a description of the various sensory aspects of the observed action (Rizzolatti & Sinigaglia, 2007). With respect to Theory of Mind, Rizzolatti & Sinigaglia (2007) argue that the mirror neurons indicate that intentions do not necessarily have to be represented independent of reality. That is, they are not necessarily processed independent of physical cues (see also Gallese, Cossu, & Sinigaglia, 2009). Based on the assumption that mirror neurons process the intentionality aspects of observed actions, they argue that intentions can also be processed in relation to physical cues such as motor behaviour.

Iacoboni et al. (2005) explored in an fMRI study whether the human mirror neuron system is involved in understanding the intentional aspects of a motor act. Participants were presented video clips in which they observed the same grasping action (intention condition: e.g., grasping a tea pot), which was embedded in different contexts (drinking vs cleaning). The authors reasoned that the same action done in two different contexts would represent different meanings and therefore should reflect different intentions. This intention condition was contrasted with two control conditions. In one control condition video clips were presented that depicted the different contexts without grasping actions. In the second control condition, participants had to observe context-free grasping actions. In addition to varying the intentional action, the authors manipulated the instruction. In the implicit instruction condition participants were simply required to watch the video clips. In the explicit instruction condition subjects had to attend to the objects displayed in the context condition, to the type of grip in the action condition, and they had to figure out the intention motivating the grasping action in the intention condition. Besides other brain regions within the human mirror neuron system, the lateral part of pre-SMA showed a signal increase for the intention condition compared to the context condition. In the present study, however, a signal increase was found for the medial pre-SMA for intention-based emotion attribution. This dissociation is likely due to differences in the stimulus material. In the present study the critical story information was contained in the verbal vignettes, while in the study of Iacoboni et al. (2005), the critical information was spatial (hand-grasping actions). A recent study showed that the pre-SMA is modality-specific activated: Tanaka, Honda, & Sadato (2005) revealed that the medial pre-SMA has been found to be involved in the updating of verbal material while the lateral pre-SMA has been observed to be recruited during the updating of spatial material. In addition, Iacoboni et al. (2005) observed that the medial part of the pre-SMA responded significantly to the explicit decoding of intentional actions as opposed to their passive observation. With respect to pre-SMA activity the authors argue that the pre-SMA may be involved in the controlled processing of motor intentionality.

The interpretation that the pre-SMA may play a role in the processing of intentional motor acts could be further discussed within Searle's (1983) framework, which defines intention-in-action as being opposed to prior intentions. While he defines prior intentions as intentions that are formed independent of reality cues, he supposes that intention-in-actions cannot be processed independent of physical cues, because they are defined as being bound to certain intentional actions. Since the pre-SMA seems to play a role in attributing intentions based on physical cues such as motor actions, the present results may show that during intention based emotion attribution the actor's intention may rather have been processed as an intention-in-action than as a prior intention. In other words, even adults may have processed the actor's intention rather by matching it to the outcome situation than by processing it independent of reality cues.

With respect to the role of the pre-SMA in explicitly processing motor intention, it was also found to be activated more during the observation of unintended compared to intended motor acts (Buccino et al., 2007). Although not significant, in the present study pre-SMA activity was also found to be more increased for emotion attribution based on unfulfilled (unintended) compared to fulfilled (intended) intentions (Fig. 3.3). This relative pre-SMA signal increase for unfulfilled as opposed to fulfilled intention-based emotion attributions may indicate that, in order to attribute emotions based on unfulfilled intentions, participants had to perform the intention-outcome matching strategy in a more controlled fashion than when they had to attribute emotions based on a fulfilled intention. This assumption is supported by a recent study which shows that the pre-SMA plays an important role in the inhibition of automatic motor responses (Mostofsky & Simmonds, 2008). In particular, the authors found the pre-SMA to be involved in the suppression of a prepotent or competing response and switching to a controlled response modus. In the present study, in the case of unfulfilled intentions, participants may have suppressed an automatic intention-outcome-match response based on an intention-outcome-match situation (e.g., feeling good = the intended other commonly catches the ball in a simple ball). Instead, they may have switched the automatic emotion response to a controlled intention-outcome-match strategy based on an intention-outcome mismatch situation (e.g., feeling bad = the intended other uncommonly does not catch the ball in a ball-playing game).

In sum, the activity increase in the medial pre-SMA for intention-based emotion attribution, particularly for unfulfilled intentions compared to reality judgements may index that even adult participants may have matched an 'intended situation' to an outcome situation rather than processing an actor's intention independent of reality cues. Therefore, intention-based emotion attribution, at least for neutral intentions, does not seem to require representational processes. Moreover, inferring emotions from unfulfilled intention-outcome situations seems to require the inhibition of an automatic emotion response. Therefore, particularly mismatched intention-outcomes relations seem to be processed in a controlled information processing modus.

4.2.2 Activity increase in the dorsolateral prefrontal cortex

Emotion attribution based on unfulfilled intentions, but not fulfilled intentions, was associated with an activity increase in the dorsolateral prefrontal cortex (DLPFC, BA 9). In general, the prefrontal cortex (PFC) plays an important role in the cognitive control of behaviour (for recent reviews see Badre, 2008; Badre & Wagner, 2007; Koechlin & Summerfield, 2007; Petrides, 2005). Therefore, the DLPFC activity is consistent with the assumption that the processing of a mismatch in intention-outcome relations may be associated with controlled information processing.

With respect to cognitive-control theories the PFC is assumed to exert its control by maintaining and biasing task-relevant information over competing task-irrelevant information and to exert this control hierarchically along a rostral-caudal axis (Badre, 2008; Koechlin & Summerfield, 2007). The more rostral a brain region is located along this axis, the more abstract its control demands are supposed to be. For example, Badre & D'Esposito (2007) tested whether the functional gradient along the caudal to rostral axis of the PFC is based on a representational hierarchy that is supposed to be ranked by the abstractness of the representation to be selected. These results could help further specify the role of the DLPFC in processing abstract representations. The authors defined a representation to be more abstract than another representation to the extent that it generalizes over specific categories. That is, a more abstract or superordinate representation was defined as comprising a category or class of categories of subordinate representations. Based on this hierarchical definition of abstractness, the authors presented tasks that started at the lowest level from the concrete motor response (first-order abstraction level). At this first-order abstraction task the relational operation was to map competing simple perceptual cues to a specific motor response (response task; cues: coloured squares). At the second-order abstraction task, the relational operation was to map competing cues that were more complex than the simple perceptual cues from the response task to a predefined motor response (feature task; cues: objects in coloured squares). At the third-order abstraction task the relational operation was to map competing relational properties between two objects to a predefined motor response (dimension task; cues: two objects in coloured squares). The context task at the fourth-order abstraction level was identical to the dimension task. The frequency, however, with which a colour-to-dimension mapping occurred, was varied. While at the first- and second-order abstraction task the cue-to-response mapping was more stimulus-driven, at the third- and fourth-order abstraction tasks, the cue-to-response mapping was based on more stimulus-independent operations, such as relational properties between objects. The authors observed the hypothesised hierarchical PFC organisation along a rostral-caudal axis: The dorsal premotor cortex was sensitive to the first-order abstraction level and the anterior dorsal premotor cortex was involved in processing tasks on a second-order abstraction level. Interestingly, the DLPFC was activated for the third-order abstraction task, and, finally, the frontal polar cortex was observed to be sensitive to the fourth-order abstraction task. Concerning the DLPFC and the frontal polar cortex, Badre & D'Esposito's (2007) findings first show that these brain regions are involved in more stimulus-independent operations. Second, these findings show that the frontal pole is to a greater degree involved in processing abstract representations than the DLPFC.

Based on Badre & D'Esposito's (2007) findings on the involvement of the DLPFC in processing abstract, stimulus-independent operations, two interpretations can be derived with respect to the DLPFC activity increase for emotions inferred from unfulfilled intentions. First, the DLPFC activity may indicate that, in addition to more concrete, outcome oriented information processes, as indexed by the pre-SMA activity, emotion attribution based on unfulfilled intentions may require more abstract, stimulus-independent operations. Second, as argued above, the frontal pole, to a greater degree as the DLPFC, is supposed to be involved in computing abstract relational operations (for review see Ramnani & Owen, 2004). While inferring emotions from unfulfilled intentions was associated with DLPFC activity, false belief reasoning as opposed to true belief reasoning was found to be associated with frontal pole activity (Sommer et al., 2007). Therefore, relative to false belief reasoning, emotion attribution based on unfulfilled intentions may require less abstract stimulus-independent operations.

More specifically with respect to the DLPFC involvement in abstract stimulus-independent operations, the DLPFC plays an important role in processing abstract mental operations required during executive processing, particularly the manipulation of information in working memory (Owen, McMillan, Laird, & Bullmore, 2005; Wager & Smith, 2003). The DLPFC activity for emotion attribution based on unfulfilled intentions may therefore indicate that the stimulus-independent processes participants had performed may have been based on a higher need of manipulating information in working memory than during reality judgements. This seems reasonable because during emotion attribution inferred from unfulfilled intentions, the intention as well as the outcome situation had to be held in memory and had to be computed with each other. In contrast, in the reality condition, no such information manipulation was necessary. Participants only had to retrieve the second picture (e.g., 'Anna has the ball') from working memory in order to answer the reality question (e.g., 'What is Anna playing with?'). Since emotion attribution based on fulfilled intentions did not vary DLPFC activity, this result may indicated that the intended situation and the outcome situation had not been computed with one another. Instead, participants may have solely related the outcome situation to an emotion (e.g., feeling good = someone caught a ball in a ball-playing game). Regarding the DLPFC activity, there is functional overlap between emotion attribution based on unfulfilled intentions and false belief reasoning because false belief relative to true belief understanding was also observed to be associated with DLPFC activity (Sommer et al., 2007).

In sum, the present results show that emotions inferred from intention-outcome relations, particularly mismatching intention-outcome relations, may be associated both with stimulus-dependent processes, as indexed by the pre-SMA activity, and with stimulus-independent processes, as indexed by the DLPFC activity. Whereas with respect to false belief reasoning, intention-based emotion attribution seems to be based on less demanding abstract operations than false belief reasoning. The manipulation of information in working memory is likely underlying these stimulus-independent operations, as indexed by the DLPFC activity. Working memory operations, therefore, seem to be a common operation required both during emotion attribution based on unfulfilled intentions and false belief reasoning.

Furthermore, an fMRI study by Lau, Rogers, Haggard, & Passingham (2004) showed that there seems to be a special coupling of the DLPFC and the pre-SMA during the controlled processing of intentional information. In this study participants had to perform the temporal judgment task developed by Libet, Gleason, Wright, & Pearl (1983). In the intention condition participants were required to pay attention to their intention before the movement. They were required to report the timing of their intention to move. In contrast, in the control condition subjects had to report when they had actually pressed the button. While the pacing of the actions and the amount of time for preparation was similar across conditions, the two temporal judgments differed significantly. Based on these findings the authors reasoned that the participants were genuinely attending to different events. The pre-SMA, together with the DLPFC and the lateral superior parietal cortex, were the only brain regions that responded significantly to intention processing. In a connectivity analysis, the authors observed that the activity between the pre-SMA and the DLPFC increased significantly from the movement to the intention condition, but not with respect to the pre-SMA and the parietal activation. Based on these findings, the authors suggest that there is a special functional relationship between the pre-SMA and the DLPFC activity during the attention to intentions.

4.2.3 Activity increase in the ventrolateral prefrontal cortex

Besides pre-SMA and DLPFC activity, emotion attribution based on unfulfilled intentions was associated with activity in the ventrolateral prefrontal cortex (VLPFC), particularly the anterior VLPFC (BA 47). The VLPFC plays an important role in the cognitive control of memory (Badre & Wagner, 2007). While the anterior VLPFC is supposed to be involved in the controlled access to stored conceptual representations, the mid-VLPFC (BA 45) is argued to support a domain-general selection process that operates post-retrieval to resolve competition among active representations. Therefore, the present findings suggest that during emotion attribution for unfulfilled intentions, scripts may have been retrieved in a controlled information processing modus (e.g., 'people feel sad when their intentions mismatch the state of reality'). This interpretation is consistent with empirical evidence on VLPFC activity in association with the retrieval of emotional information, such as affective faces (Nakamura et al., 1999) or the coupling of affective faces and emotional situations (Sommer, Döhnel, Meinhardt, & Hajak, 2008). Moreover, the findings suggest that emotion attribution based on both an unfulfilled intention and on false belief understanding require script retrieval, because false belief relative to true belief understanding was also observed to be associated with BA 47 activity (Sommer et al., 2007).

4.2.4 Activity decrease in the orbital part of the paracingulate cortex

Besides activity increases in the pre-SMA and the lateral prefrontal cortex, intention-based emotion attribution, particularly for unfulfilled intentions, was associated with a linear activity decrease in the orbital part of the paracingulate cortex (BA 32), which is part of the ventromedial prefrontal cortex. Specifically, emotion attribution based on unfulfilled intentions showed the strongest decrease in functional activity followed by a lesser decrease in functional activity for emotions inferred from fulfilled intentions. In contrast, the reality condition was associated with an activity increase, compared to both the baseline level and to the intention conditions.

The signal decrease observed for intention based emotion attribution may be explained within the framework of the 'default mode network'. The 'default mode network' comprises brain regions within cortical midline structures, including the ventromedial prefrontal cortex (Buckner, Andrews-Hanna, & Schacter, 2008; Gusnard, Raichle, & Raichle, 2001; Raichle et al., 2001). Neuroimaging studies observed functional deactivations in 'default mode network' related brain regions when subjects were engaged in active task processing. Moreover, these task-induced deactivations were related to decreasing self-referential processes (McKiernan, D'Angelo, Kaufman, & Binder, 2006). For example, McKiernan et al. (2006) explored the relationship between task difficulty, task-unrelated thoughts and task-induced deactivations. First, the authors observed that with increasing task difficulty in an exogenous task, task-unrelated thoughts decreased. Further, as task-induced deactivations increased, task-unrelated thought declined. Therefore, deactivations within the 'default mode network' are commonly interpreted as a disengagement of self-referential processes towards task-related processes (for reviews see Beer, 2007; Northoff & Bermpohl, 2004). That VMPFC activity decreases are likely associated with the suspension of task-unrelated, internally triggered, affective thoughts in favour of task-related, cognitive processes could be shown in a study by Gusnard, Akbudak, Shulman, & Raichle (2001). The authors explored the involvement of the medial prefrontal cortex in self-referential mental activity, cued by affective pictures. In the internally cued, self-referential condition, participants had to perform pleasantness judgements. In the externally cued, non self-referential condition, participants had to perform indoor-outdoor judgements on the affective material. The authors observed a dissociation in the medial PFC. While the DMPFC was associated with an activity increase for the control condition over the self-referential condition, both conditions were related with activity decreases in the VMPFC, particularly the self-referential condition that was based on affective self-referential judgements. These findings can be interpreted that internal, affective processes are suspended in the VMPFC in order to process external cues. Further support for the involvement of the VMPFC in emotional processing comes from empirical evidence showing an MPFC dissociation with respect to cognitive versus affective processing. While the DMPFC has been shown to be mainly involved in cognitive processing, the VMPFC has been found to play an important role in emotional processing (Ochsner, Hughes, Robertson, Cooper, & Gabrieli, 2008; Steele & Lawrie, 2004). Based on these findings it can be argued that intention-based emotion attribution, particularly for unfulfilled intentions, seems to be associated with the suspension of task-unrelated, internally triggered, affective thoughts in favour of task-related, cognitive processes, as indexed by the activity increases in brain regions associated with more cognitive processes such as the pre-SMA and the dorso- and ventrolateral prefrontal cortex.

Which internally triggered, affective processes may have to be suspended in favour of task performance? The orbital MPFC (oMPFC) is involved in the representation and updating of possible future outcomes, that is, the evaluation of personal outcome values (Amodio & Frith, 2006; Rushworth, Behrens, Rudebeck, & Walton, 2007). For example, Knutson, Taylor, Kaufman, Peterson, & Glover (2005) observed that oMPFC activity was associated with the anticipated gain probability, and Walton, Devlin, & Rushworth (2004) found that oMPFC activity varied with the need to monitor the outcomes of externally guided actions. To interpret the activity increase associated with reward processing in terms of the default network, reward processing could be argued to be a highly self-referential process, and hence should result in signal increases within the 'default mode network'. Based on this assumption, signal decreases would be expected in the oMPFC when processing others' reward. The present study found oMPFC signal decreases associated with emotion attribution based on attributing emotions to others. Moreover, a linear relationship between task demands and task-induced deactivations was observed. To integrate the 'default mode network' account and the reward account, the observed oMPFC deactivation may indicate that when task demands increase, which seems to be mostly the case for emotion attribution based on unfulfilled intentions, as indexed by the strongest task-induced deactivation for these emotion judgements, affective processes concerning ones own reward in situations like that may be suspended in order to represent and update the reward value of other's outcome situations.

4.3 Summary

The present study aimed to specify the information processes that may underlie emotion attribution based on intention-outcome-relations, an ability that shortly develops before the ability to understand false belief scenarios. It was hypothesized that inferring emotions from intention-outcome-relations would be associated with both distinct and common neural networks with respect to false belief understanding. Specifically, it was predicted that frontal brain regions, particularly the DMPFC, would be associated with intention-based emotion attribution. Furthermore, it was predicted that more posterior brain regions, particularly the TPJ, would be less associated with intention-based emotion attribution. Both predictions were confirmed. These results, on the one hand, confirm the hypothesis that the medial prefrontal cortex (MPFC) is recruited as well for intention-based emotion attribution as for false belief understanding. On the other hand, however, the neuroimaging findings show that distinct subregions within the MPFC are associated with intention-based emotion attribution and false belief understanding. While false belief reasoning has been shown to be associated with activity in more rostral parts of the MPFC (Aichhorn et al., 2008a; Fletcher et al., 1995; Gallagher et al., 2000; Perner et al., 2006; Saxe & Kanwisher, 2003; Saxe & Powell, 2006; Saxe et al., 2006; Saxe & Wexler, 2005; Sommer et al., 2007), the present results reveal that intention-based emotion attribution seems to be associated with activity in more posterior parts of the MPFC, specifically the medial pre-SMA. Moreover, emotion attribution based on intention-outcome-relations varies activity in the orbital part of the paracingulate cortex, which, in turn, is not commonly recruited during false belief understanding. These results suggest that, although the MPFC is recruited during both intention-based emotion attribution and false belief understanding, the story seems to be more complex in that intention-based emotion attribution is probably associated with distinct information processes compared to false belief reasoning. Understanding false beliefs is supposed to require a representational understanding of mental states because false beliefs have to be evaluated independent of reality cues. Neuroimaging findings suggest a special role of the rostral MPFC and the TPJ in false belief understanding. Hence, these brain regions are supposed to be associated with the representational understanding of mental states. With respect to intention-based emotion attribution, neither the rostral MPFC nor the TPJ were found to be activated. Therefore, the results suggest that emotions can be inferred from intention-outcome relations without representing the actor's intention independent of reality. Specifically, the pre-SMA activity observed during intention-based emotion attribution supports developmental theories which assume that even adults may infer emotions from intention-outcome relations by matching others' intentions in relation to the outcome situation rather than processing the intention independent of reality cues. That is, adults take an objective stance rather than a subjective stance in intention-based emotion attribution. Besides stimulus-dependent processes, stimulus-independent processes seem to particularly underlie emotion attribution based on unfulfilled intentions. These processes are likely to be the manipulation of information in working memory, as indexed by the DLPFC activity, and script retrieval, as indexed by the VLPFC activity. Both operations seem to be basic processes required both during emotion attribution based on unfulfilled intentions and on false belief reasoning. Moreover, emotion attribution based on unfulfilled intentions may be particularly associated with a suspension of self-referential, reward related outcome evaluations in favour of representing and updating others' possible future outcomes, as indexed by the oMPFC activity decrease.

Based on the results of the first experiment, the second experiment explores the neural network associated with emotions inferred from the integration of immoral intentions into intention-outcome-relations, an ability which is acquired shortly after the development of false belief understanding.

5. INTRODUCTION

STUDY II
EMOTIONS INFERRED FROM THE INTEGRATION OF IMMORAL INTENTIONS INTO INTENTION-OUTCOME-RELATIONS

While the first experiment was concerned with the neural correlates associated with emotion attribution based on intention-outcome-relations, the second experiment aims at investigating brain regions that process the integration of immoral intentions into the processing of intention-outcome-relations. Before the age of six children have difficulties to appropriately perform this integration process. That is, so called happy victimizer attributions are observed in children beyond six years (chapter 5.1). The developmental chapter is followed by neuroimaging findings on the processing of transgression scenarios (chapter 5.2). The introduction concludes with a summary of the introduction part and with deducing the research question (chapter 5.3).

5.1 The happy victimizer phenomenon

The happy victimizer phenomenon is defined as a developmental shift around the age of 6 to 7 in young children's judgments of a victimizer's emotions in response to a transgression or willpower scenario. Though children before age 6 to 7 are able to understand moral values, compared to older children and adults they judge victimizers to feel more positive and less negative emotions after successful transgression, and 'moral heros' to feel less positive and more negative emotions after the potential transgressor has restrained from the transgression (Arsenio, Gold, & Adams, 2006; Arsenio & Kramer, 1992; Arsenio & Lover, 1995; Barden, Zelko, Duncan, & Masters, 1980; Keller, Gummerum, Wang, & Lindsey, 2004; Keller, Lourenco, Malti, & Saalbach, 2003; Lagattuta, 2005; Lourenco, 1997; Nunner-Winkler & Sodian, 1988; Sokol, 2004; Sokol & Chandler, 2004; Yuill et al., 1996).

Nunner-Winkler & Sodian (1988) were the first who systematically explored the happy victimizer phenomenon (for earlier findings see Barden et al., 1980). In their first experiment out of a series of three experiments, Nunner-Winkler & Sodian (1988) presented 4- to 8-year-olds stories of a child transgressing (immoral version) and a child sustaining from transgression (moral version). All age groups understood the moral rule that it is not right to transgress. Interestingly, in the immoral version younger children compared to older children judged a victimizer to feel less negative and more positive emotions (positive emotion attributions: 74% in 4-year-olds, 40% in 6-year-olds; negative emotion attributions: 90% in 8-year-olds). Further, in the moral version, where the protagonist resisted to transgress, the authors observed more 'sad moral hero' responses in 6-year-olds compared to 8-year-olds (for similar 'sad moral hero' findings see Lagattuta, 2005). With respect to children's justifications of their emotion attribution responses, Nunner-Winkler & Sodian (1988) observed an age effect with more outcome-oriented justifications among 4-year-olds to more morally-oriented responses to 8-year-olds. In addition to the emotion attribution task, the authors conducted a moral judgement task in which the children were required to judge the moral worth of two victimizers who differed in their emotional reactions in response to successful transgression (feeling happy versus feeling sorry). Interestingly, while 4-year-olds' moral judgements did not differ whether a transgressor was feeling happy or sorry after his transgression, 6- and 8-year-olds judged the happy victimizer to be worse than the sorry victimizer. In their second and third experiment the authors confirmed the robustness of the happy victimizer pattern in younger children. In their second experiment 5-year-olds showed the happy victimizer pattern even after moral aspects had been made salient (e.g., the victim's physical harm, the victimizer's tangible profit). Moreover, in their third experiment the authors confirmed their hypothesis that young children's happy victimizer responses are restricted to situations where there is a conflict between personal motives and moral standards. In the unintentional harm done by a neutral actor condition, where there is no conflict between personal motive and moral standards, 5-year-olds appropriately judged the character as not being bad, but as feeling bad. Interestingly, in the intentional harm done by ill-motivated actor condition, where there is a conflict between the personal immoral motive and the moral standard, 5-year-olds judged the transgressor as being bad, but as feeling good. Based on younger children's happy victimizer responses, Nunner-Winkler & Sodian (1988) reasoned that, although even young children understand moral rules, they do not seem to integrate their moral knowledge into situations where there is a conflict between personal goals (to get what one wants) and moral rules (not to transgress). Further, the authors argue that younger children's attribution of positive feelings to the victimizer and negative feelings to the 'moral hero' primarily seem to be a function of the goal-oriented satisfaction of the victimizer's interests. This hypothesis is supported by findings from Wiersma & Laupa (2000) who found no happy victimizer effect in 3- to 5-year-olds in scenarios where a person transgresses without an explicitly specified goal. Moreover, Nunner-Winkler & Sodian (1988) argued that older children's attribution of negative feelings to the transgressor and positive feelings to the 'moral hero' is a function of more morally-oriented considerations.

Subsequent research on the happy victimizer phenomenon showed that the attributional reversal from younger children's happy victimizer responses to older children's sad victimizer responses observed in earlier studies (Barden et al., 1980; Nunner-Winkler & Sodian, 1988) turned out to be more complex and subtle. For example, several subsequent studies revealed that for primary emotion responses (e.g., 'How does [the victimizer] feel?') the happy victimizer responses had been shown to be based predominately on goal-oriented considerations for younger as well as for older children (Arsenio & Kramer, 1992; Lagattuta, 2005; Lourenco, 1997; Sokol, 2004; Sokol & Chandler, 2004; Yuill et al., 1996), and had been observed to persist even into adolescence and adulthood (Lagattuta, 2005; Murgatroyd & Robinson, 1993; Murgatroyd & Robinson, 1997). Interestingly, primary emotion responses had been shown to vary with the interview procedure (Sokol, 2004; Sokol & Chandler, 2004; Yuill et al., 1996). For example, Sokol and colleagues (2004) showed that when the interview procedure focused on more goal-oriented aspects (e.g., 'How does [the victimizer] feel?'), as is the case in the traditional interview procedure on the happy victimizer research, all 5- to 7-year-olds' primary emotion judgements revealed happy victimizer responses. In contrast, when the interview focused more on moral aspects (e.g., 'How does [the victimizer] feel about acting like that?'), 5- to 7-year-olds judged the victimizer to feel sad as their primary emotion response. Not only are primary emotion responses affected by the interview procedure, but also adolescents' primary emotion attributions with respect to the self (e.g., 'Imagine you did what [the victimizer] did. How would you feel afterwards?') were observed to be a function of social desirability responses (Krettenauer & Eichler, 2006).

While primary emotion responses have shown to be a function of the interview procedure and of social desirability considerations, secondary emotion responses (e.g., 'What else does [the victimizer] feel?') had turned out to rather robustly measure the happy victimizer phenomenon in young children (Arsenio & Kramer, 1992; Lagattuta, 2005; Lourenco, 1997; Sokol, 2004; Sokol & Chandler, 2004; Yuill et al., 1996). For example, Arsenio & Kramer (1992) were the first who integrated a secondary emotion probe into their interview protocol. While for the first emotion probe the majority of 4- to 8-year-olds gave happy victimizer responses based on predominately goal-oriented considerations, for the secondary emotion probe the authors observed an age effect. While the majority of the 4-year-olds persisted to give happy victimizer responses also when they had the opportunity to further reflect on the victimizer's feelings, 6- and 8-year-olds compared to 4-year-olds provided significantly more opposite valenced, moral emotions (e.g., the victimizer feels sad). Furthermore, the attributional shift from happy to sad victimizer responses were not as sharp as was observed in the early research on the happy victimizer phenomenon. While the majority of the 8-year-olds provided moral emotion responses when probed with the least directive probe (e.g. 'Do you think the actor could be feeling anything else?'), the majority of the 6-year-olds justified the victimizer to feel sad for the most directive probe question (e.g., 'You said your friend [the victimizer] would be happy when he got your swing. What if he looked at you on the ground and saw that you were very sad, could he feel anything else besides happy?'). Arsenio & Kramer (1992) concluded that there seems to be a more subtle shift from 4-year-olds' judgements that victimizers are simply happy to 8-year-olds' tendency to view victimizers as feeling more mixed or conflicting emotions. Further evidence that children's secondary emotion responses are a more valid measure for detecting age related changes in their happy victimizer responses comes from Sokol's (2004) doctoral thesis, who observed significant relationships between cognitive processes that may underlie the happy victimizer responses only when taking into account the children's secondary emotion responses.

A recent study explored the happy victimizer phenomenon in greater detail and extended research to prohibitive rule situations (Lagattuta, 2005). First, the author compared 4- to 7-year-olds' emotion predictions and explanations with adult responses in both transgression and willpower trials. Second, responses in prohibitive rule scenarios were compared with emotion predictions and explanations in simple, rule-free situations where a neutral desire was either fulfilled or unfulfilled. Third, in addition to the trials where participants had to predict and explain a character's feelings (predict-and-explain-trials), Lagattuta (2005) presented trials where participants had to provide explanations for a character's feelings in response to transgression and willpower situations (explain-only-trials). Fourth, connections between emotion predictions and emotion explanations were assessed.

With respect to emotion attribution in transgression trials, Lagattuta (2005) showed that also in prohibitive rule scenarios there is an attributional shift from positive emotions to mixed emotions between 4 and 7 years. Moreover, while in willpower scenarios 5-year-olds reported more 'sad moral hero' emotions; 7-year-olds attributed more mixed emotions. Further, the author also showed that for the primary emotion response not only the majority of children but also almost all adults attributed positive emotions to transgression trials and negative emotions to willpower scenes. In contrast, for the secondary emotion probe only from seven years on significantly more mixed emotions were reported. With respect to emotion explanations, there was no age effect for goal-oriented justifications. However, for rule-oriented (e.g., 'Because he listened to the rule') and future-oriented explanations (e.g., 'Because she might have gotten hurt if she had done it.') a developmental effect was observed. Rule-oriented explanations were significantly more often provided by 7-year-olds and adults compared to 4- and 5-year-olds. Interestingly, 7-year-olds provided future-oriented explanations more often than did any other age group. Moreover, most of the future-oriented explanations focused on possible negative outcomes for the self or potential negative outcomes for others rather than references with respect to harm or punishment.

In addition to transgression trials, Lagattuta (2005) included simple desire stories. With respect to emotional intensity ratings four- and five-year-olds, as with 7-year-olds and adults, predicted that a person whose desire was fulfilled in no-rule scenarios would feel significantly better than those whose desire was fulfilled in the transgression trials. Furthermore, four- and five-year-olds, as with 7-year-olds and adults, judged a character to feel significantly worse in rule-free situations where its desire has been blocked than in moral situations where the character has chosen to refrain from desire fulfilment. These results show that, although younger children do not seem to be able to provide mixed emotion responses to transgressors and willpower actors, they seem to have some first insight that the basic relationship between neutral desires and emotions (e.g., goal fulfilment = feeling good; goal-blocked = feeling bad) is modified by rule considerations.

In addition to transgression vignettes where participants had to predict and explain the transgressor's emotion, Lagattuta (2005) hypothesized that the inclusion of predict-only-trials would make it easier for younger children to integrate the influence of rule considerations into their justifications for transgression and willpower judgements. This was the case for 5-year-olds' rule-oriented explanations. That is, 5-year-olds provided significantly more rule-oriented explanations when they were asked to explain why a character is feeling sad after transgression and why he is feeling good after willpower behaviour than when they had to both predict and explain the character's feelings. Interestingly, 4-year-olds did not profit from this explanation-only method. Moreover, the combined explanations for both the predict-and-explain and the explain-only trials showed that 4-year-olds compared 7-year olds and adults provided significantly more goal-oriented explanations.

Finally, Lagattuta (2005) assessed the connections between emotion predictions and emotion explanations. Children and adults showed a consistent link between emotion prediction and explanation type, even when controlled for age. That is, more rule- and future-oriented explanations were provided when a transgressor was judged to feel bad and a 'moral hero' to feel good than when the transgressor was judged to feel good and the 'moral hero' to feel sad. Furthermore, children and adults explained emotions in relation to characters' goals more often after desire-outcome match than after desire-outcome mismatch trials.

In sum, Lagattuta (2005) generalizes previous research findings on the happy victimizer phenomenon to prohibitive rule situations by showing that children under 7 years are impaired in attributing mixed emotions to transgressors and willpower actors. Moreover, she showed that, although goal-oriented explanations were predominately observed even in the adult sample, 4-year-olds provided significantly more goal-oriented explanations than 7-year-olds and adults. Interestingly, she observed that despite their deficits, even young children seem to have some knowledge with respect to the fact that rule considerations can decrease the emotional intensity to which a person feels happy in transgression situations and to which a character feels sad in 'moral hero scenarios', compared to simple rule-free scenarios. Moreover, 5-year-olds, but not 4-year-olds, are able to provide twice as many rule-oriented explanations when they had to explain a character's feelings than when they had to predict and explain it.

While Lagattuta (2005) extended the happy victimizer research to prohibitive rule situations, another recent study explored cultural effects on the happy victimizer phenomenon by comparing German with Portuguese children (Keller et al., 2003). In addition, the authors investigated whether happy victimizer responses are a function of whether emotions had to be attributed to the victimizer or to the self (e.g., 'How would you feel if you had done that?'). First, the authors observed a main effect of culture on the emotions attributed both to the self and the victimizer. German children attributed more negative emotions than Portuguese children both to the self and to the victimizer. Second, the authors observed an age-related self-other split in emotion attribution. Although both 5-year-olds and 8-year-olds attributed more negative emotions to the self than to the victimizer, older children compared to younger children attributed more negative emotions to both the self and the victimizer. The finding on the self-other-split, however, has to be interpreted with caution because, at least for the older children, the self-other differentiation observed in emotion judgements during victimizer scenarios could also be a function of social desirability responses (Krettenauer & Eichler, 2006).

While most researchers on the happy victimizer phenomenon have speculated about the specific nature of the cognitive constraints that may underlie younger children's inability to provide mixed emotions in situations where one's personal desire conflicts with moral standards, only few have directly tested possible underlying constraints. Arsenio & Lover (1995) have speculated that young children's inability to attribute conflicting emotions to a victimizer may be a function of an immature Theory of Mind development (also see Astington, 2004). This assumption has been tested in several recent studies (Baird & Astington, 2004; Sokol, 2004; Sokol & Chandler, 2004; Sokol et al., 2004). For example, in his doctoral thesis Sokol (2004; also see Sokol & Chandler, 2004) observed a relationship between young children's happy victimizer responses and the development of an interpretive ToM understanding. In addition to the false belief task, ToM development can be measured by tasks that vary in their interpretational complexity (Lalonde & Chandler, 2002). As suggested by Sodian & Thoermer (2006), a more simple interpretive ToM understanding is supposed to require one to understand that a person who has false information about reality will interpret reality falsely, as measured by the false belief task. In contrast, a more complex interpretative ToM understanding is supposed to require one to understand that identical reality information can be interpreted differently from different perspectives, as measured by the droodle task which only allows a restricted view on reality ('droodle-task': e.g., a restricted view on the picture depicting 'a ship arriving too late to save a drowning witch'). While a more simple interpretive ToM understanding develops between 4- to 5-years, a more complex interpretative

ToM understanding develops at the age of 6 to 7 years. Coming back to Sokol (2004), he observed that the development of an interpretive ToM understanding, as measured by the droodle task, is a function of attributing mixed emotions to victimizers. When controlled for age, children with an interpretive ToM understanding were more likely to attribute mixed victimizer emotions. That the development of an interpretative ToM understanding was a significant predictor for judging a victimizer to feel mixed emotions, was further supported by the fact that the age by ToM correlation, when controlled for emotion attribution, remained significant, but not the age by emotion attribution, when the ToM factor was partialled out. Interestingly, in the non happy-victimizer condition, emotion attribution and ToM development no longer correlated when controlled for age. That ToM development is an important predictor for attributing mixed emotions to victimizers is further supported by another study from Sokol et al. (2004). They presented 5- to 7-year-olds a series of slapstick films, in which a puppet character named Punch attempts to harm another character named Judy. The films depicted two attempted, but failed, murder scenes, in which Punch had every intention of harming Judy. Both interpretive and non-interpretive children adequately responded to questions about Punch's subversive intention. However, when controlled for age, children with an interpretive ToM, as measured by the droodle task, rated Punch's action as significantly more harshly than non-interpretive children.

The studies from Sokol and colleagues show that the development of an interpretive ToM understanding predicts the attribution of mixed emotions to victimizers. More evidence on young children's inability to interpret the same reality cue differently comes from another recent study (Baird & Astington, 2004). The authors tested 4- to 7-year-olds' ability to evaluate the same action (e.g., two characters turning on a hose) differently in relation to the actor's intention (bad motive condition: e.g., 'Susan's brother had built a sand castle in the backyard, and Susan wanted the sand castle to collapse'; neutral motive condition: e.g., 'Jessica's mother had planted some seeds in the backyard, and Jessica wanted to help take care of the garden'). Interestingly, 4-year-olds were significantly worse than both 5- and 7-year-olds at differentiating the character's actions in terms of moral quality. In contrast, 5- and 7-year-olds were equally skilled at assigning different moral evaluations to characters performing identical actions. Furthermore, 4-year-olds were significantly worse than both 5- and 7-year-olds at differentiating the character's actions in terms of punishment ratings. In contrast, 5- and 7-year-olds were equally skilled in their punishment ratings. In addition, when controlled for age, the authors observed a positive correlation between children's false belief understanding and their ability to differently evaluate the same action with respect to moral parameters and punishment ratings.

In sum, research on the happy victimizer phenomenon shows that around the age of 6 to 7 years there is a subtle, developmental change from providing happy victimizer responses to providing more mixed emotions to victimizer. This change, however, is not as sharp as was observed in early research. Children as well as adults show a goal-oriented happy victimizer pattern as their primary emotion response. Before age 6 to 7, however, when asked to provide additional emotion responses, children predominately pertain to the happy victimizer responses. Above this age children and adults provide more mixed emotions based on more morally-oriented, rule-oriented, and future-oriented responses. Furthermore, young children's happy victimizer responses seem to be a general phenomenon since it has been shown not only in transgression but also in willpower scenarios, and not only in physical harm situations, but also in other situations such as stealing, lying, and prohibitive-rule situations. In addition, more recent research has shown that young children's inability to attribute mixed feelings to victimizers is likely a function of an immature interpretive ToM understanding. However, whether false belief understanding and emotion attribution based on integrating moral considerations into intention-outcome-relations is associated with common or different neural networks remains to be explored.

5.2 Neuroimaging findings on the processing of transgression scenarios

By now, the majority of neuroimaging studies on moral reasoning have concentrated on the neural network associated with the processing of moral dilemmas (Greene & Haidt, 2002; Greene, Sommerville, Nystrom, Darley, & Cohen, 2001; Heekeren, Wartenburger, Schmidt, Schwintowski, & Villringer, 2003; Schaich, Hynes, Van, Grafton, & Sinnott-Armstrong, 2006), immoral statements (Moll, Oliveira-Souza, Bramati, & Grafman, 2002; Takahashi et al., 2004), pictures (Moll et al., 2002), or scripts (Shin et al., 2000). Therefore, this is the first neuroimaging study which explores the brain regions implicated in emotion attribution based on integrating other's immoral intentions into intention-outcome-relations. Thereby, this study particularly focuses on the investigation of brain regions implicated in the processing of mixed emotions inferred from fulfilled moral transgression scenarios. Currently, three studies have investigated the neural correlates associated with self-attributed moral emotions in transgression scenarios (Berthoz, Armony, Blair, & Dolan, 2002; Finger, Marsh, Kamel, Mitchell, & Blair, 2006; Kedia, Berthoz, Wessa, Hilton, & Martinot, 2008). Out of these three studies, only Berthoz et al. (2002) and Finger et al. (2006) aimed at exploring brain regions associated with emotion attribution inferred from intended compared to unintended transgression. For example, Berthoz et al. (2002) showed that the processing of statements depicting intentional versus unintentional social transgressions was associated with activity in the rostral part of the medial prefrontal cortex, the dorsal part of the anterior cingulate and paracingulate cortex, the superior prefrontal cortex including the premotor cortex, and the inferior parietal cortex. Further, Finger et al. (2006) observed that intentional moral transgression compared to unintentional social transgression was associated with activity in the dorsal part of the medial prefrontal cortex (DMPFC), the dorso- and ventrolateral prefrontal cortex, the premotor cortex and the temporal cortex. However, the results of the Finger et al. (2006) study have to be interpreted with caution because the intention and the transgression factor are confounded. In sum, results of both studies suggest that self-attributed emotions based on intentional versus unintentional transgression seem to be associated with activity in the prefrontal cortex, particularly the dorsal and rostral part of the medial prefrontal cortex as well as premotor brain regions.

Because the ability to reason about false beliefs and the ability to integrate moral considerations into the processing of intention-outcome-relations have been observed to be developmentally closely connected, a recent fMRI study investigated the neural network involved in the interaction between false belief reasoning and moral judgements in intention-outcome-scenarios (Young, Cushman, Hauser, & Saxe, 2007). The authors presented scenarios where an immoral actor behaved based on either a true or false belief about reality. In the true belief scenario, the victimizer's immoral intention was related to a negative outcome (intended harm). In the false belief scenario, its immoral intention was related to a positive outcome (attempted harm). Actors that held a neutral intention also acted based on either a true or false belief about reality. While in the true belief scenarios, the character's neutral behaviour resulted in a positive outcome (no-harm), in the false belief scenes its neutral behaviour resulted in a negative outcome (unintended harm). Intention by outcome interactions were analysed in functional ROIs in those brain regions supposed to be associated with belief reasoning, as was measured by a false belief versus false photograph contrast. The authors observed that the right temporo-parietal-junction (RTPJ) and the DMPFC showed an activity increase for moral judgements based on attempted harm compared to intended harm and compared to no-harm vignettes (for similar results see Young & Saxe, 2008). These findings suggest that brain regions implicated in false belief reasoning seem to be recruited for moral judgements in those cases where a victimizer's behaviour was based on a false belief about reality as in the attempted harm trials. In contrast, when a victimizer's behaviour was based on a true belief, as in the intended harm scenarios, the DMPFC and the RTPJ seem to be less associated with the processing of moral transgression. These findings, however, do not support other results which show DMPFC activity during emotion attribution also in cases where a victimizer fulfills its immoral intention based on a true belief about reality (Berthoz et al., 2002; Finger et al., 2006). The diverging findings could be due to differences in analysis methods (fROI analysis versus whole brain analysis). Further, the divergence could be due to differences with respect to the tasks: self-related emotion attributions (Berthoz et al., 2002; Finger et al., 2006) versus other-related moral judgements (Young et al., 2007). Alternatively, the diverging findings could also be due to differences in the salience of the intention-outcome-relation. While in the studies of Berthoz et al.

(2002) and Finger et al. (2006) the intention-outcome-relation was not made explicit, in the study of Young et al. (2007) the intention-outcome-relation was made explicit.

5.3 Summary and research question

The first study explored emotion attribution based on intention-outcome-relations. To go a step further on exploring intention-based emotion attribution, the present study is the first that investigates the neural network involved in emotion attribution based on the integration of an actor's immoral intention into intention-outcome-relations. Interestingly, this ability develops after the ability to attribute emotions inferred from intention-outcome-relations and it even follows the development of false belief understanding.

Based on developmental findings on the happy victimizer phenomenon, it is hypothesised that particularly for fulfilled immoral intentions adults would give mixed emotion responses. Further, it is hypothesised that similar information processes would be associated with emotion attribution based on immoral intentions relative to emotion attribution based on neutral intentions. Based on the findings from experiment 1, particularly premotor brain regions, along with the dorso- and ventrolateral prefrontal cortex, as well as the ventromedial prefrontal cortex are predicted to be recruited during emotion attribution based on this integration process. Beyond, developmental evidence suggests that the ability for emotion attribution based on integrating immoral intentions into intention-outcome-relations is a function of a developing ToM understanding. This finding is reflected on neuroimaging level because brain regions that are implicated in ToM, particularly the DMPFC, have been observed to be also involved in emotion attribution based on transgression scenarios. Therefore, it is predicted that emotion attribution based on the integration of immoral intentions into intention-outcome-relations would also be associated with activity in the DMPFC.

To explore emotion attribution based on immoral intentions, cartoon stories with verbal vignettes were presented. The material was adopted from developmental studies on the happy victimizer phenomenon (Yuill et al., 1996). The nonverbal material was held equivalent across the experimental conditions, which only differed in their verbal vignettes. A 2 by 2 factorial design was used. The factor 'intention' varied on whether the protagonist held a neutral or immoral intention. The factor 'intention-outcome-relation' varied on whether the protagonist's intention matched or mismatched the outcome situation. Besides the emotion attribution conditions, a non-mental control condition was used that solely described physical processes.

6. METHODS

STUDY II
EMOTIONS INFERRED FROM THE INTEGRATION OF IMMORAL INTENTIONS INTO INTENTION-OUTCOME-RELATIONS

6.1 Participants

Eighteen right-handed subjects (10 females, 8 males, age range = 18-20 years, M = 19.44 years, SD = .78 years) with no neurological or psychiatric history participated in the study. All gave informed consent according to the guidelines of the local Ethic Committee.

6.2 Task and material

Analogous to experiment 1, intention-based emotion attribution was explored by a modified, fMRI compatible version adopted from the developmental study of Yuill et al. (1996). Cartoons were presented which were described by verbal vignettes. The nonverbal pictures depicted three children playing, a protagonist and two recipients (Figs. 6.1 to 6.3). Eight story contexts were used: children playing with a ball, a teddy, a balloon, a toy airplane, a toy duck, a toy car, badminton, or hockey. The nonverbal material was held equivalent across the study conditions, which only differed in their verbal vignettes. For the emotion attribution conditions a 2 x 2 factorial design was used with the within subject factors 'intention' (neutral intention, immoral intention) and 'intention-outcome-relation' (match: Fulfilled Intention, mismatch: Unfulfilled Intention). The factor 'intention-outcome-relation' varied on whether the protagonist's intention matched (fulfilled intention) or mismatched the outcome situation (unfulfilled intention). The intention factor varied on whether the protagonist held a neutral (Fig. 6.1) or immoral intention (Fig. 6.2). Besides emotion attribution conditions, a non-mental control condition (Non-Ment) was used that solely described physical processes (Fig. 6.3).

In the emotion attribution conditions, the verbal vignette in the first story picture described the protagonist's intention (neutral intention: e.g. 'Max wants to throw the ball to Lena'; immoral intention: e.g. 'Max wants to hurt Lena with the ball'). The second story picture presented the outcome of the intended action (fulfilled neutral intention: e.g., 'Max throws the ball to Lena'; unfulfilled neutral intention: e.g., 'Max throws the ball to Paul'; fulfilled immoral intention: e.g. 'Max hurts Lena with the ball'; unfulfilled immoral intention: e.g. 'Max hurts Paul with the ball'). In the third picture the protagonist was depicted and the participants were instructed to reason about the protagonist's emotion dependent on its prior intention and on the outcome of the intended actions (e.g., 'How does Max feel?'). To separate reasoning about the actor's emotion from giving a motor response, participants were instructed not to respond before the response stimulus was presented. The response stimulus depicted two smileys (positive, negative). Responses were given by pressing a button.

In the reality condition verbal vignettes in the first two pictures described the scene (e.g., picture 1: 'The kids are playing with the puck'; picture 2: 'Max has the puck'). In the third picture participants were instructed to reason about the toy the kids were playing with ('What is Lena playing with?'). In the response stimulus the target toy was presented along with one distracter toys. Here, participants were instructed to respond to the target toy by pressing a button.

For each condition 20 trials were presented. Stimulus complexity was held equivalent across conditions. The protagonist's and the recipients' gender was counterbalanced, as well as the protagonist's presentation side on the screen (left/right). All children were presented without a facial expression in order not to trigger specific emotion attribution processes by the visual input. In the response trials the presentation order of the smileys and of the toys was counterbalanced.

In order to obtain more specific emotion attribution responses, a rating task was conducted following the scanning session (Appendix B). In the rating task the same cartoon-stories were presented as during the fMRI session and the same emotion attribution conditions were used. In each emotion attribution condition four to five trials were presented. Participants were instructed to rate the actor's emotion on eight emotion dimensions (happiness, pride, satisfaction, schadenfreude, surprise, embarrassment, sadness, anger). Each dimension varied on a five-point Likert scale ranging from 1 (not at all) to 5 (very strong).

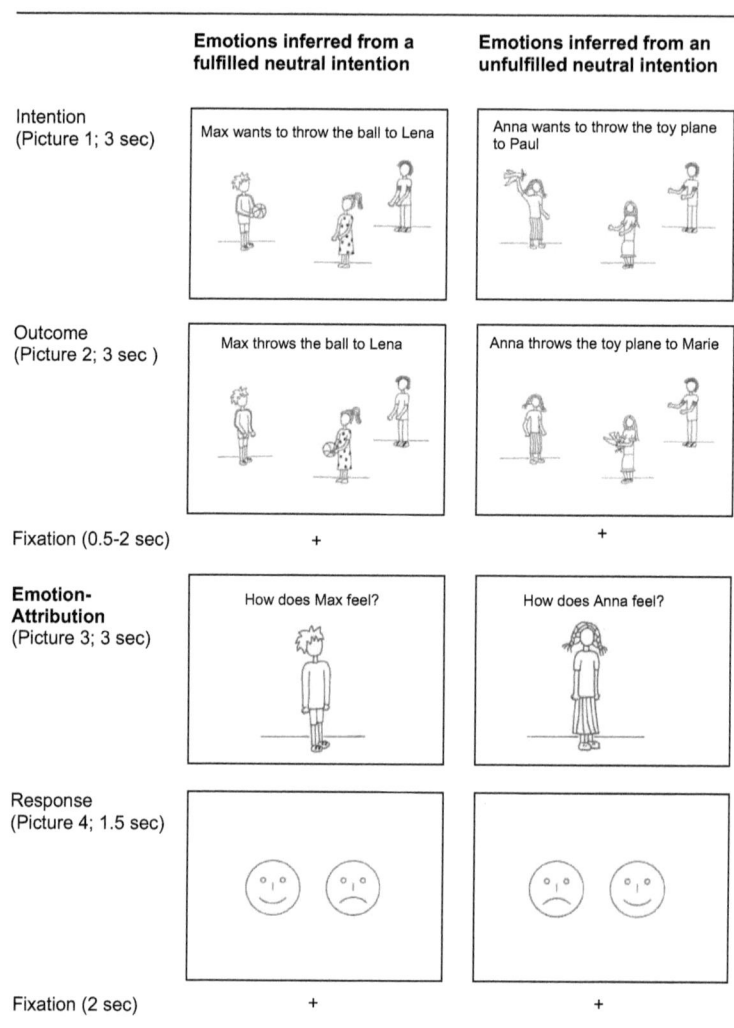

Fig. 6.1: Example of emotions inferred from a fulfilled neutral intention (left) and an unfulfilled neutral intention (right). Pictures were consecutively presented with intermediate fixation periods varying in time intervals. Functional analysis focused on the emotion attribution stimuli (picture 3).

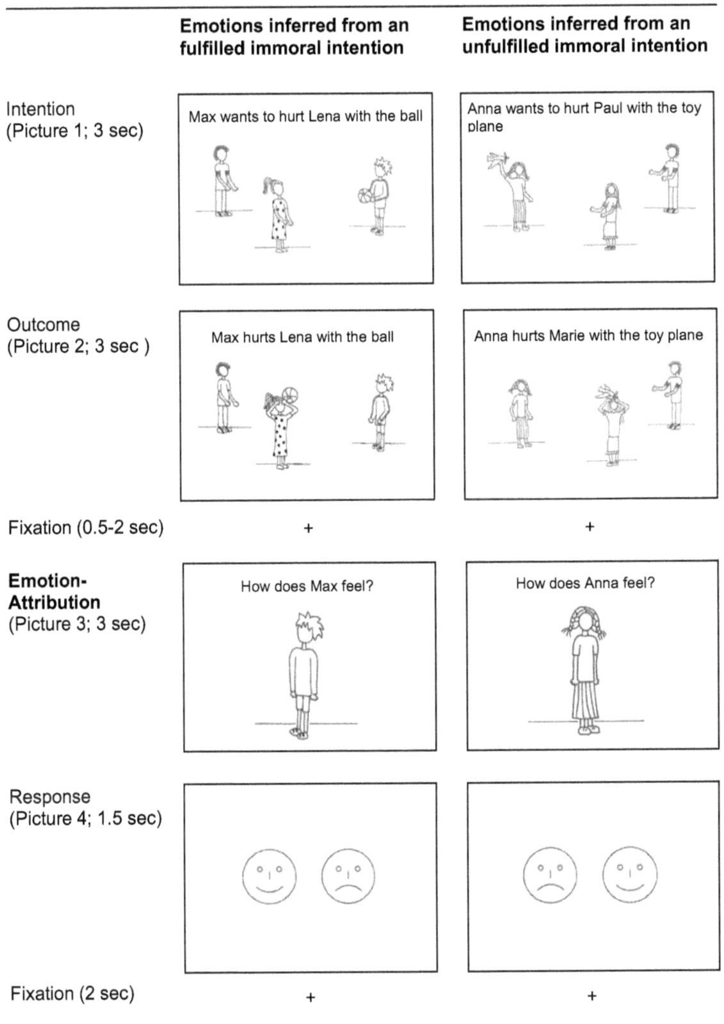

Study II – Methods

	Emotions inferred from an fulfilled immoral intention	Emotions inferred from an unfulfilled immoral intention
Intention (Picture 1; 3 sec)	Max wants to hurt Lena with the ball	Anna wants to hurt Paul with the toy plane
Outcome (Picture 2; 3 sec)	Max hurts Lena with the ball	Anna hurts Marie with the toy plane
Fixation (0.5-2 sec)	+	+
Emotion-Attribution (Picture 3; 3 sec)	How does Max feel?	How does Anna feel?
Response (Picture 4; 1.5 sec)		
Fixation (2 sec)	+	+

Fig. 6.2: Example of emotions inferred from a fulfilled immoral intention (left) and an unfulfilled immoral intention (right). Pictures were consecutively presented with intermediate fixation periods varying in time intervals. Functional analysis focused on the emotion attribution stimuli (picture 3).

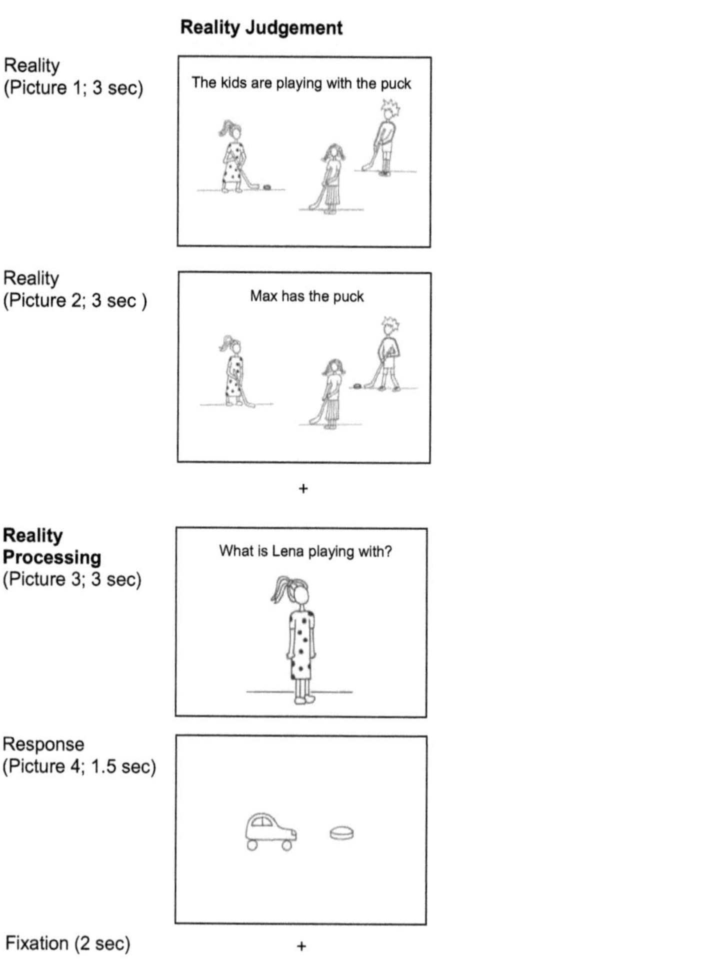

Reality Judgement

Reality
(Picture 1; 3 sec)   The kids are playing with the puck

Reality
(Picture 2; 3 sec)   Max has the puck

+

Reality Processing
(Picture 3; 3 sec)   What is Lena playing with?

Response
(Picture 4; 1.5 sec)

Fixation (2 sec)   +

Fig. 6.3: Example of a reality judgement trial. Pictures were consecutively presented with intermediate fixation periods varying in time intervals. Functional analysis focused on the reality processing stimuli (picture 3).

6.3 Experimental procedure

Prior to the experimental task participants attended a training session to become familiar with the stimulus material. Following the fMRI session the rating task was conducted. During the fMRI session stimuli were back-projected onto a screen. Foam padding restricted head motion. The experimental conditions were randomly presented across the scanning session. Within each trial stimuli were presented in a fixed order: the story stimuli (pictures 1 and 2) were presented for 3 seconds each. The emotion attribution stimulus and the reality processing stimulus (picture 3) were presented for 3 seconds each. The response stimulus (picture 4) was presented for 1.5 seconds. Fixation periods were presented before each trial (2 sec) and before the third picture (0.5-2 sec). Fixation periods were included to measure an inter-stimulus baseline and to properly model the hemodynamic response function associated with emotion attribution. Presentation software was used for stimulus presentation and for response recording (Neurobehavioral Systems Inc., Albany, CA). Responses were recorded by using two buttons of a five-button fMRI compatible response pad (LUMItouch, Photon Control Inc., Burnaby, Canada).

6.4 Statistical analysis of the behavioural data

The statistical analysis of the behavioural data was conducted with SPSS 15. In the reality condition response accuracy (in percentage) was analysed. With respect to the emotion attribution responses obtained during the scanning session, for every emotion dimension (positive, negative) the mean percentage of emotion responses out of its total amount was calculated. In the rating task for every emotion dimension (happiness, pride, satisfaction, schadenfreude, surprise, embarrassment, sadness, anger) a mean rating score ranging from 1 (not at all) to 5 (very strong) was computed. On every emotion dimension statistical analysis was done by conducting a repeated measurement Analysis of Variance (ANOVA) with a 2 x 2 factorial design: 'intention' (neutral intention, immoral intention) x 'intention-outcome-relation' (match: fulfilled intention, mismatch: unfulfilled intention). Further statistical analysis was done by post-hoc paired t-tests with Greenhouse-Geisser alpha-correction. T-tests were two-tailed and a value of $p \leq .05$ was used to determine statistical significance.

6.5 Imaging and image preprocessing

Scanning was performed in an interleaved fashion on a 3 Tesla fMRI scanner (Siemens Allegra, Erlangen, Germany). The functional images sensitive to blood oxygenation level dependent (BOLD) contrasts were acquired by $T2^*$-weighted echo planar images (EPI, TR = 2.82 sec, TE = 50 ms, flip angle = 90°, in plane matrix 64 x 64, FoV = 192 mm). The images consisted of 32 axial slices with 3mm thickness and 3 x 3mm in plane resolution. During the scanning 494 volumes were acquired. High resolution structural weighted images (TR = 2.25 sec, TE = 2.6 ms, TI = 900 ms, voxel size 1x1x1mm, 160 axial slices, FoV = 256 mm) were recorded from all participants. The scanning session lasted approximately 30 min.

All images were preprocessed using the SPM5 software package (http://www.fil.ion.ucl.ac.uk/spm/), which is based on MATLAB 7.0 software (The MathWorks Inc., Natick, MA). For each participant functional images were slice-timed corrected using the middle slice as reference, realigned to the first volume by rigid body transformation to correct for participants' motion, normalised to the Montreal Neurological Institute (MNI) reference brain (Collins et al., 1994), and spatially smoothed by a Gaussian kernel with a full-width half-maximum of 8 mm.

6.6 Statistical analysis of the images

All statistical first and second-level analysis were conducted with the SPM5 software package and were based on the entire brain. The analysis focused on amplitude changes in the hemodynamic response function (HRF) associated with emotion attribution and reality judgement (picture 3). Fixation periods served to measure an inter-stimulus baseline and to analyse the hemodynamic response function associated with emotion attribution and reality judgement.

In the first-level analysis a fixed effects analysis was computed for each participant based on the general linear model (GLM). The stimuli were modelled by boxcars of 3 seconds, which were then convolved with the HRF, along with its time and dispersion derivatives to account for any temporal and spatial shifts in the response of the stimuli (Friston et al., 1998). Also included were six covariates to capture residual movement-related artefacts, and a single covariate representing the mean (constant) over scans. The data were high-pass filtered with a frequency cutoff at 128 seconds. Statistical parametric maps (SPMs) were generated for each subject by t-statistics derived from contrasts utilizing the HRF (Friston et al., 2002). The derivates from the statistical model were not included in the contrasts.

First, these contrasts of interest were computed on the individual analysis level for **emotion attribution compared to reality judgements:**

Contrast 1: Emotions inferred from fulfilled neutral intentions versus reality judgement ('Fulfilled Neutral Intention' versus 'Non-Ment')

Contrast 2: Emotions inferred from unfulfilled neutral intentions versus reality judgement ('Unfulfilled Neutral Intention' versus 'Non-Ment')

Contrast 3: Emotions inferred from fulfilled immoral intentions versus reality judgement ('Fulfilled Immoral Intention' versus 'Non-Ment')

Contrast 4: Emotions inferred from unfulfilled immoral intentions versus reality judgement ('Unfulfilled Immoral Intention' versus 'Non-Ment');

Second, these contrasts of interest were computed on the individual analysis level for the **main effects** of the factor 'intention' and 'intention-outcome relation':

Contrast 5: Emotions inferred from immoral versus neutral intentions ('Fulfilled Immoral Intention' + 'Unfulfilled Immoral Intention' versus 'Fulfilled Neutral Intention' + 'Unfulfilled Neutral Intention')

Contrast 6: Emotions inferred from unfulfilled versus fulfilled intentions ('Unfulfilled Neutral Intention' + 'Unfulfilled Immoral Intention' versus 'Fulfilled Neutral Intention' + 'Fulfilled Immoral Intention')

Finally, these contrasts of interest were computed on the individual analysis level for **emotion attribution dependent on the factors intention and intention-outcome-relation:**

Contrast 7: Emotions inferred from unfulfilled neutral intentions versus fulfilled neutral intentions ('Unfulfilled Neutral Intention' versus 'Fulfilled Neutral Intention')

Contrast 8: Emotions inferred from unfulfilled immoral intentions versus fulfilled immoral intention ('Unfulfilled Immoral Intention' versus 'Fulfilled Immoral Intention')

Contrast 9: Emotions inferred from fulfilled immoral intentions versus fulfilled neutral intentions ('Fulfilled Immoral Intention' versus 'Fulfilled Neutral Intention')

Contrast 10: Emotions inferred from unfulfilled immoral intentions versus unfulfilled neutral intentions ('Unfulfilled Immoral Intention' versus 'Unfulfilled Neutral Intention')

These single-subject first-level contrast images from the weighted beta-images were introduced into second-level random-effects analysis to allow for population inference. One-sample t-tests were computed to assess functional activity associated with emotion attribution compared to reality judgements (contrasts 1 to 4), as well as for the main effects of the factors 'intention' (contrast 5) and 'intention-outcome-relation' (contrast 6). This study was specifically interested in brain regions showing an 'intention' by 'intention-outcome-relation' interaction effect. To test for interaction effects, a one-way ANOVA (including non-sphericity correction) was computed including contrasts 1 to 4. Within this ANOVA, an F-contrast was computed to test for brain regions showing a significant interaction effect (Henson & Penny, 2003). Interaction effects were further analysed by one-sample t-tests (contrasts 7 to 10). All fMRI results reported here are based on voxel statistics computed with SPM for the entire brain. The resulting set of significant voxel values for each contrast constituted an SPM map. The maps were thresholded at $T = 3.79$ ($p \leq .001$ uncorrected), overlaid on the MNI template, and labelled by using the MNI coordinates. For graphical purposes, in those brain regions showing significant effects, mean cluster values (parameter estimates) were extracted by using the SPM5 software.

7. RESULTS

STUDY II
EMOTIONS INFERRED FROM THE INTEGRATION OF IMMORAL INTENTIONS INTO INTENTION-OUTCOME-RELATIONS

7.1 Behavioural findings

The emotion attribution results obtained during the fMRI session are shown in Tables 7.1 and 7.2, as well as in Figure 7.1. Mean accuracy for the reality judgement was 93 % (SD = 3.5 %). The ANOVA on the factors 'intention' and 'intention-outcome-relation' showed a significant interaction effect ($F(1,17)$ = 5.69, $p \leq .05$), and a main effect of 'intention-outcome-relation' ($F(1,17)$ = 313.72, $p \leq .001$). No main effect of 'intention' was observed ($F(1,17)$ = 3.65, n.s.). Regarding the main effect of 'intention-outcome-relation', more positive and less negative emotions were attributed after intention-outcome-match trials compared to intention-outcome-mismatch trials (Tab. 7.1). This main effect was qualified by a significant 'intention' by 'intention-outcome-relation' interaction effect (Tab. 7.2, Fig. 7.1). Post-hoc t-tests on the interaction effect revealed that more positive and less negative emotions were attributed following a fulfilled neutral intention compared to a fulfilled immoral intention ($t(13)$ = 2.20, $p \leq .05$,), as well as following a fulfilled neutral intention compared to a unfulfilled neutral intention, and a fulfilled immoral intention compared to an unfulfilled immoral intention (Fulfilled Neutral Intention versus Unfulfilled Neutral Intention: $t(17)$ = 25.41, $p \leq .001$; Fulfilled Immoral Intention versus Unfulfilled Immoral Intention: $t(17)$ = 12.64, $p \leq .001$). In other words, the interaction results demonstrate that subjects attributed the greatest amount of positive emotions to fulfilled neutral intentions and the greatest amount of negative emotions to scenarios depicting an unintended harm (unfulfilled immoral intention). That is, on the one hand in the case of intended victimization (fulfilled immoral intention) less positive emotions compared to non-harming fulfilled intentions were attributed. On the other hand, however, subjects attributed more positive emotions to intended victimization as opposed to unintended harm trials.

Table 7.1: Mean emotion attribution scores of the fMRI session in the intention and in the intention-outcome-relation condition.

Emotion[a]	Intention				Intention-Outcome-Relation			
	Neutral Intention		Immoral Intention		Fulfilled		Unfulfilled	
	M	(SD)	M	(SD)	M	(SD)	M	(SD)
Positive	54	(7)	45	(12)	91	(12)	8	(9)
Negative	46	(7)	55	(12)	9	(12)	92	(9)

Notes: M, mean; SD, standard deviation.
[a] Percentage of negative and positive responses out of the total amount of emotion responses

Table 7.2: Mean emotion attribution scores of the fMRI session dependent on the factor intention (neutral intention, immoral intention) and intention-outcome-relation (match: fulfilled intention, mismatch: unfulfilled intention).

Emotion[a]	Neutral Intention				Immoral Intention			
	Fulfilled		Unfulfilled		Fulfilled		Unfulfilled	
	M	(SD)	M	(SD)	M	(SD)	M	(SD)
Positive	97	(3)	10	(14)	84	(24)	6	(8)
Negative	3	(3)	90	(14)	16	(24)	94	(8)

Notes: M, mean; SD, standard deviation.
[a] Percentage of negative and positive responses out of the total amount of emotion responses

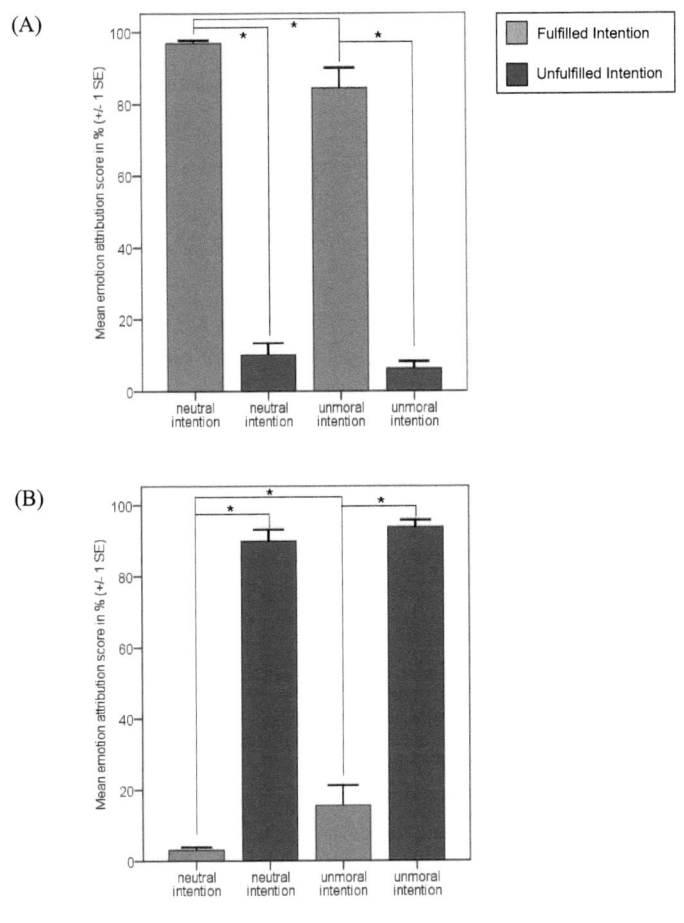

Fig. 7.1: Mean emotion attribution scores (+/- 1 SE) obtained during the fMRI session. Intention by intention-outcome-relation interaction effects were observed for positive (A) and negative (B) emotions.

More specific emotion attribution results were obtained during the rating task that followed the fMRI session (Tabs. 7.3 to 7.6, Figs. 7.2 to 7.4). Emotion ratings were obtained from the emotions happiness, pride, satisfaction, schadenfreude, surprise, embarrassment, sadness, and anger. Rating scores ranged from 1 (not at all) to 5 (very strong). All emotions showed a main effect of 'intention-outcome-relation' (Tab. 7.3 and 7.5, Fig. 7.2A). More happiness, pride, satisfaction, and schadenfreude were attributed after intention-outcome-match trials than intention-outcome-mismatch trials. In contrast, more surprise, embarrassment, sadness, and anger were attributed following intention-outcome mismatch trials compared to intention-outcome match trials. Moreover, all emotions except surprise and anger showed a main effect of intention (Tab. 7.3 and 7.5, Fig. 7.2B). For immoral compared to neutral intentions less happiness, pride, and satisfaction, and more embarrassment (Fig. 7.3A), sadness (Fig. 7.3B), but also more schadenfreude were attributed. Furthermore, for the emotions happiness, pride, satisfaction, and schadenfreude main effects were qualified by intention x intention-outcome-relation interaction effects (Tab. 7.5 and 7.4, Fig. 7.4). Post-hoc t-tests showed that more happiness, pride, and satisfaction were attributed following a fulfilled neutral intention compared to a fulfilled immoral intention, as well as following a fulfilled neutral intention compared to an unfulfilled neutral intention, and a fulfilled immoral intention compared to an unfulfilled immoral intention (Tab. 7.6, Fig. 7.4A-C). In other words, for the emotions happiness, pride and satisfaction the rating results revealed a similar pattern as for the behavioural results obtained during the fMRI session. Subjects attributed the greatest intensity of these emotions to fulfilled neutral intentions and the least intensity to unfulfilled immoral intentions. That is, on the one hand in the case of intended victimization (fulfilled immoral intentions) less happiness, pride, and satisfaction were attributed as opposed to non-harming fulfilled intentions. On the other hand, however, subjects attributed significantly more happiness, pride, and satisfaction to intended victimization compared to unintended harm trials. Moreover, the interaction effect on the immoral emotion schadenfreude revealed that schadenfreude was attributed significantly more often following intended victimization compared to both non-harming trials and unintended victimization scenarios (Tab. 7.6, Fig. 7.4D).

Study II – Results

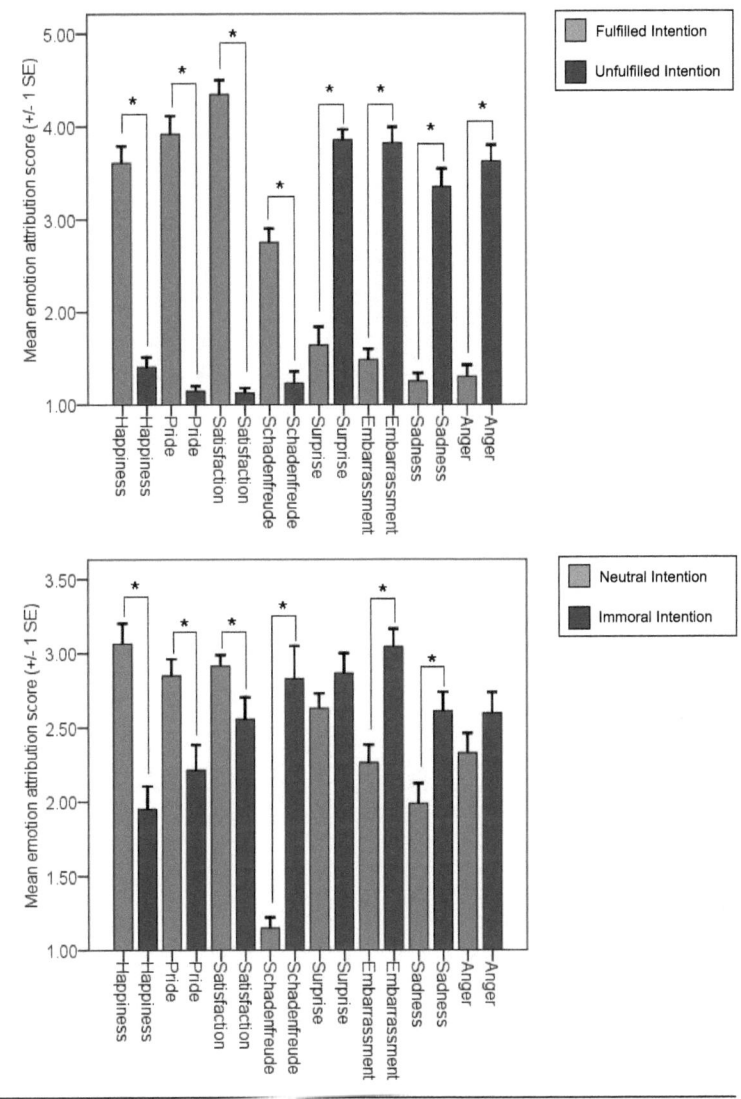

Fig.7.2: Main effects of the factors intention-outcome relation (A) and intention (B) in the rating task. Rating scores range from 1 (not at all) to 5 (very strong).

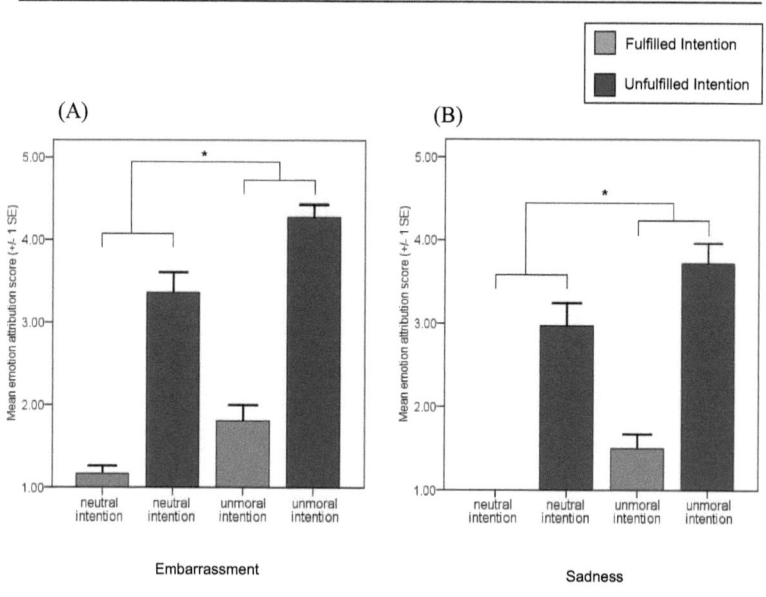

Fig. 7.3: Main effects of intention in the rating task for embarrassment (A) and sadness (B). Rating scores range from 1 (not at all) to 5 (very strong).

Study II – Results

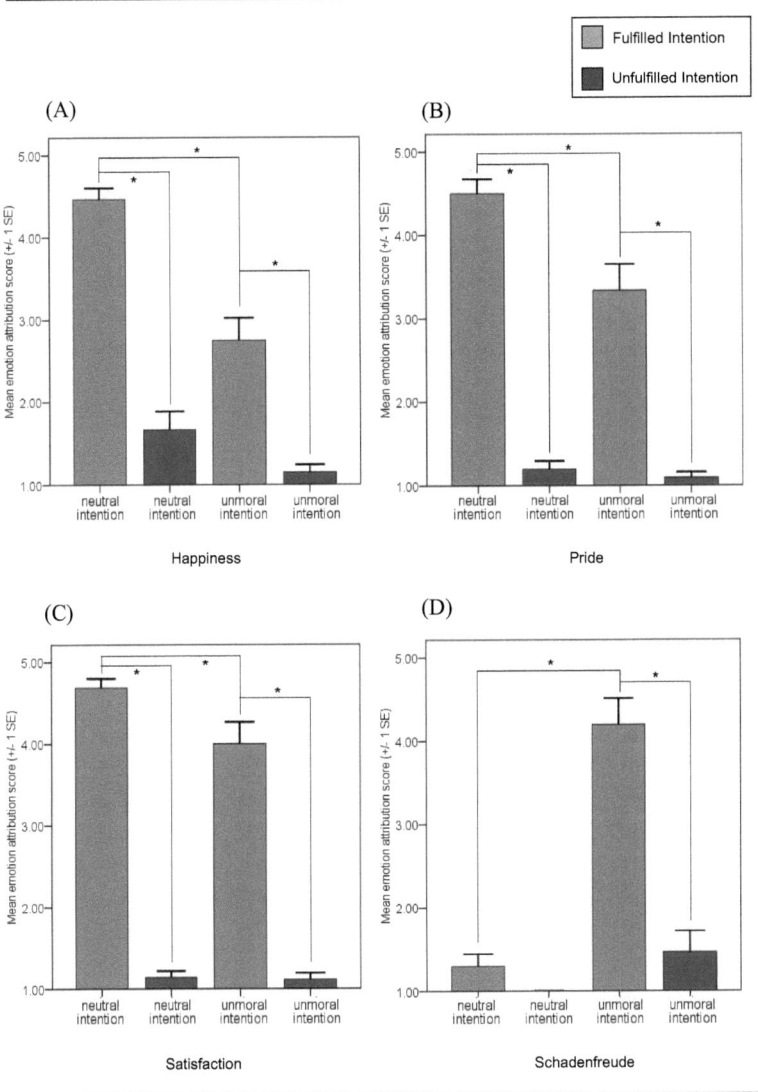

Fig. 7.4: Intention by intention-outcome relation interaction effects in the rating task. Rating scores range from 1 (not at all) to 5 (very strong).

Table 7.3: Mean emotion attribution scores of the rating task in the intention and in the intention-outcome-relation condition.

Emotion[a]	Intention				Intention-Outcome-Relation			
	Neutral Intention		Immoral Intention		Fulfilled		Unfulfilled	
	M	(SD)	M	(SD)	M	(SD)	M	(SD)
Happiness	3.06	(.59)	1.95	(.66)	3.61	(.77)	1.41	(.46)
Pride	2.85	(.48)	2.21	(.73)	3.92	(.83)	1.14	(.23)
Satisfaction	2.91	(.32)	2.56	(.63)	4.34	(.67)	1.13	(.22)
Schadenfreude	1.15	(.31)	2.83	(.93)	2.75	(.65)	1.23	(.54)
Surprise	2.63	(.42)	2.86	(.57)	1.64	(.83)	3.85	(.48)
Embarrassment	2.26	(.51)	3.04	(.52)	1.49	(.49)	3.82	(.73)
Sadness	1.99	(.58)	2.61	(.54)	1.25	(.36)	3.35	(.83)
Anger	2.33	(.57)	2.60	(.59)	1.30	(.53)	3.63	(.72)

Notes: M, mean; SD, standard deviation.
[a] Emotion ratings ranging from 1 (not at all) to 5 (very strong).

Table 7.4: Mean emotion attribution scores of the rating task dependent on the factors intention (neutral intention, immoral intention) and intention-outcome-relation (match: fulfilled intention, mismatch: unfulfilled intention).

Emotion[a]	Neutral Intention				Immoral Intention			
	Fulfilled		Unfulfilled		Fulfilled		Unfulfilled	
	M	(SD)	M	(SD)	M	(SD)	M	(SD)
Happiness	4.46	(0.60)	1.67	(0.94)	2.75	(1.15)	1.15	(0.38)
Pride	4.50	(0.73)	1.19	(0.42)	3.33	(1.34)	1.09	(0.27)
Satisfaction	4.68	(0.49)	1.14	(0.33)	4.00	(1.14)	1.11	(0.34)
Schadenfreude	1.30	(0.63)	1.00	(0.00)	4.19	(1.34)	1.46	(1.07)
Surprise	1.59	(0.88)	3.67	(0.66)	1.69	(0.89)	4.04	(0.64)
Embarrassment	1.17	(0.40)	3.36	(1.04)	1.81	(0.81)	4.28	(0.65)
Sadness	1.00	(0.00)	2.97	(1.16)	1.50	(0.73)	3.72	(1.02)
Anger	1.07	(0.31)	3.58	(1.02)	1.53	(0.93)	3.67	(0.82)

Notes: M, mean; SD, standard deviation.
[a] Emotion ratings ranging from 1 (not at all) to 5 (very strong).

Table 7.5: ANOVA for the emotion attribution results from the rating task.

Emotion	F-value (df = 1, 17)	p-value
Happiness		
Intention	34.76	$\leq .001$
Intention-Outcome-Relation	125.18	$\leq .001$
Intention x Intention-Outcome-Relation	13.98	$\leq .01$
Pride		
Intention	11.45	$\leq .01$
Intention-Outcome-Relation	226.27	$\leq .001$
Intention x Intention-Outcome-Relation	11.19	$\leq .01$
Satisfaction		
Intention	4.47	$\leq .05$
Intention-Outcome-Relation	353.01	$\leq .001$
Intention x Intention-Outcome-Relation	7.79	$\leq .05$
Schadenfreude		
Intention	45.68	$\leq .001$
Intention-Outcome-Relation	68.96	$\leq .001$
Intention x Intention-Outcome-Relation	32.76	$\leq .001$
Surprise		
Intention	3.04	n.s.
Intention-Outcome-Relation	74.60	$\leq .001$
Intention x Intention-Outcome-Relation	1.33	n.s.
Embarrassment		
Intention	27.37	$\leq .001$
Intention-Outcome-Relation	109.95	$\leq .001$
Intention x Intention-Outcome-Relation	.96	n.s.
Sadness		
Intention	13.88	$\leq .01$
Intention-Outcome-Relation	87.92	$\leq .001$
Intention x Intention-Outcome-Relation	.372	n.s.
Anger		
Intention	2.71	n.s.
Intention-Outcome-Relation	130.07	$\leq .001$
Intention x Intention-Outcome-Relation	1.03	n.s.

Table 7.6: Post-hoc t-test results on the rating task to further analyse intention by intention-outcome-relation interaction effects.

Emotion	t-value (df = 17)	p-value
Happiness		
Fulfilled Neutral Intention vs Fulfilled Immoral Intention	3.60	$\leq .01$
Unfulfilled Neutral Intention vs Unfulfilled Immoral Intention	.80	n.s.
Fulfilled Neutral Intention vs Unfulfilled Neutral Intention	19.56	$\leq .001$
Fulfilled Immoral Intention vs Unfulfilled Immoral Intention	7.47	$\leq .001$
Pride		
Fulfilled Neutral Intention vs Fulfilled Immoral Intention	7.31	$\leq .001$
Unfulfilled Neutral Intention vs Unfulfilled Immoral Intention	1.20	n.s.
Fulfilled Neutral Intention vs Unfulfilled Neutral Intention	11.38	$\leq .001$
Fulfilled Immoral Intention vs Unfulfilled Immoral Intention	6.15	$\leq .001$
Satisfaction		
Fulfilled Neutral Intention vs Fulfilled Immoral Intention	2.59	$\leq .05$
Unfulfilled Neutral Intention vs Unfulfilled Immoral Intention	.23	n.s.
Fulfilled Neutral Intention vs Unfulfilled Neutral Intention	27.47	$\leq .001$
Fulfilled Immoral Intention vs Unfulfilled Immoral Intention	10.94	$\leq .001$
Schadenfreude		
Fulfilled Neutral Intention vs Fulfilled Immoral Intention	7.48	$\leq .001$
Unfulfilled Neutral Intention vs Unfulfilled Immoral Intention	1.83	n.s.
Fulfilled Neutral Intention vs Unfulfilled Neutral Intention	2.01	n.s.
Fulfilled Immoral Intention vs Unfulfilled Immoral Intention	7.43	$\leq .001$

7.2 Neuroimaging findings

FMRI results are listed in Tables 7.7 to 7.10 and are shown in Figures 7.5 to 7.7. With respect to emotions inferred from neutral intentions, the results from the first experiment were mainly confirmed. That is, particularly emotions inferred from unfulfilled neutral intentions compared to reality judgements were associated with a signal increase in the medial part of the pre-supplementary motor area (pre-SMA, BA 6), as well as the left dorsolateral (DLPFC, BA 9) and left ventrolateral prefrontal cortex (VLPFC, BA 47, Tab. 7.7). With respect to emotions inferred from immoral intentions, specifically emotions inferred from fulfilled immoral intentions compared to reality judgements were associated with an activity increase in the medial pre-SMA, the left dorsolateral (BA 9) and the left ventrolateral prefrontal cortex (BA 47), as well as a brain region at the transition between the right insula and the right ventrolateral prefrontal cortex (BA 13/45, Tab. 7.7). Emotions inferred from unfulfilled immoral intentions compared to reality judgements were associated with an activity increase in the dorsal paracingulate cortex (BA 32), the left dorsolateral (BA 9) and the left ventrolateral prefrontal cortex (BA 47), as well as the right insula (BA 13).

Table 7.7: Brain regions showing significant functional signal changes associated with emotion attribution.

Brain region	BA	Cluster Size[a]	t-value (df = 17)[b]	x,y,z (mm)[c]
Unfulfilled Neutral Intention vs Reality				
Pre-supplementary motor area	6	109	5.67[g]	14, 12, 52
Left ventrolateral prefrontal cortex	47	151	5.73[f]	-52, 18, -2
Left dorsolateral prefrontal cortex	9	237	5.50[e]	-28, 48, 38
Fulfilled Immoral Intention vs Reality				
Pre-supplementary motor area	6	592	5.70[d]	-6, 16, 64
Left ventrolateral prefrontal cortex	47	319	4.85[e]	-44, 32, -6
Left dorsolateral prefrontal cortex	9	170	4.79[f]	-28, 52, 34
Right Insula / ventrolateral prefrontal cortex	13/45	168	5.25[f]	38, 12, 8
Unfulfilled Immoral Intention vs Reality				
Dorsal paracingulate cortex	32	462	4.98[d]	8, 24, 40
Left ventrolateral prefrontal cortex	47	287	6.00[e]	-52, 18, -4
Left dorsolateral prefrontal cortex	9	233	5.65[e]	-32, 48, 34
Right Insula	13	331	7.40[d]	38, 12, 6

Notes: BA, Brodmann's areas are approximate.
[a] Numbers of activated voxels per cluster.
[b] Peak t-value in activated cluster, df = degrees of freedom.
[c] Peak coordinate of activated cluster according to the Montreal Neurological Institute (MNI) atlas.
[d] Brain region satisfies a statistical cluster threshold of $p \leq .001$ (corrected).
[e] Brain region satisfies a statistical cluster threshold of $p \leq .01$ (corrected).
[f] Brain region satisfies a statistical cluster threshold of $p \leq .05$ (corrected).
[g] Brain region satisfies a statistical cluster threshold of $p \leq .01$ (uncorrected).

Further, the main effect of intention revealed that emotions inferred from immoral compared to neutral intentions was associated with functional activity in the dorsal paracingulate cortex (BA 32, Tab. 7.8), the left ventrolateral prefrontal cortex (BA 47), and the visual cortex (BA 18/19). There was no brain region that showed a significant difference in brain activity for emotions inferred from neutral compared to immoral intentions. In addition, no brain region showed a main effect for the factor 'intention-outcome-relation'.

Table 7.8: Brain regions showing significant functional signal changes associated with the main effect of intention.

Brain region	BA	Cluster Size[a]	t-value (df = 17)[b]	x,y,z (mm)[c]
Immoral vs Neutral Intention				
Dorsal paracingulate cortex	32	314	6.28[d]	8, 38, 22
Right ventrolateral prefrontal cortex	47	148	6.53[e]	42, 20, -14
Left middle occipital cortex	19	227	5.18[d]	-50, -76, 2
Cuneus	18	133	5.42[e]	-12, -96, 10

Notes: BA, Brodmann's areas are approximate.
[a] Numbers of activated voxels per cluster.
[b] Peak t-value in activated cluster, df = degrees of freedom.
[c] Peak coordinate of activated cluster according to the Montreal Neurological Institute (MNI) atlas.
[d] Brain region satisfies a statistical cluster threshold of $p \leq .01$ (corrected).
[e] Brain region satisfies a statistical cluster threshold of $p \leq .05$ (corrected).

This study was mainly interested in brain regions showing an intention by intention-outcome-relation interaction effect. The interaction analysis showed significant effects in the pre-supplementary-motor area (pre-SMA, BA 6) and the bilateral ventrolateral prefrontal cortex (VLPFC; left: BA 47; right: BA 45, Tab. 7.9). For these brain regions the t-test analysis showed a significant signal increase associated with emotions inferred from fulfilled immoral intentions compared to fulfilled neutral intentions (Tab. 7.10; BA 6: Fig. 7.5; BA 47: Fig. 7.6; BA 45: Fig. 7.7). No other t-contrast dependent on the factors intention and intention-outcome-relation had a significant impact on functional activity in the pre-SMA and the bilateral ventrolateral prefrontal cortex.

Table 7.9: Brain regions showing significant functional signal changes associated with intention by intention-outcome relation interaction effects.

Brain region	BA	Cluster Size[a]	F-value (df = 1,85)[b]	x,y,z (mm)[c]
Pre-supplementary motor area	6	16	12.76	6, 20, 54
Right ventrolateral prefrontal cortex	45	17	13.38	54, 24, 18
Left ventrolateral prefrontal cortex	47	137	17.71	-48, 32, 2

Notes: BA, Brodmann's areas are approximate.
[a] Numbers of activated voxels per cluster.
[b] Peak t-value in activated cluster, df = degrees of freedom.
[c] Peak coordinate of activated cluster according to the Montreal Neurological Institute (MNI) atlas.

Table 7.10: Post-hoc t-test results in brain regions showing significant functional signal changes associated with the intention by intention-outcome-relation interaction.

Brain region	BA	Cluster Size[a]	t-value (df = 17)[b]	x,y,z (mm)[c]
Fulfilled Intention: Immoral vs Neutral				
Pre-supplementary motor area	6	152	5.10[d]	-4, 22, 66
Right ventrolateral prefrontal cortex	45	144	4.78[d]	54, 22, 8
Left ventrolateral prefrontal cortex	47	166	4.41[d]	-52, 18, -4

Notes: BA, Brodmann's areas are approximate.
[a] Numbers of activated voxels per cluster.
[b] Peak *t*-value in activated cluster, df = degrees of freedom.
[c] Peak coordinate of activated cluster according to the Montreal Neurological Institute (MNI) atlas.
[d] Brain region satisfies a statistical cluster threshold of $p \leq .05$ (corrected).

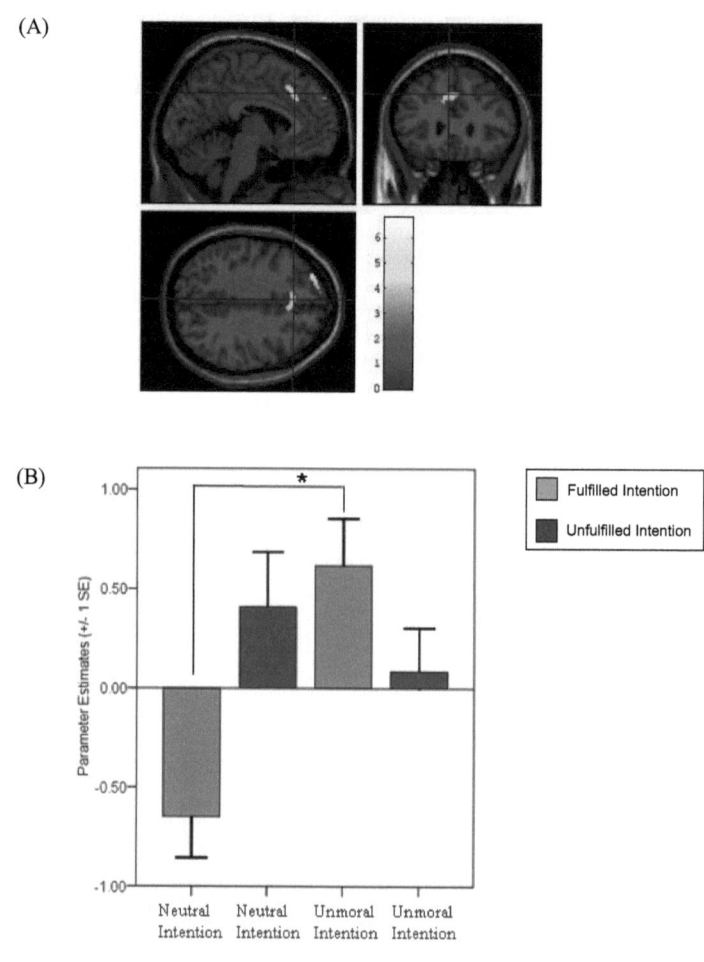

Fig. 7.5: (A) Functional changes in the amplitude of the HRF in the medial pre-supplementary motor area (BA 6) associated with an intention by intention-outcome-relation interaction effect. (B) Post-hoc t-tests showed an activity increase for fulfilled immoral compared to fulfilled neutral intentions. BA, Brodmann's areas are approximate.

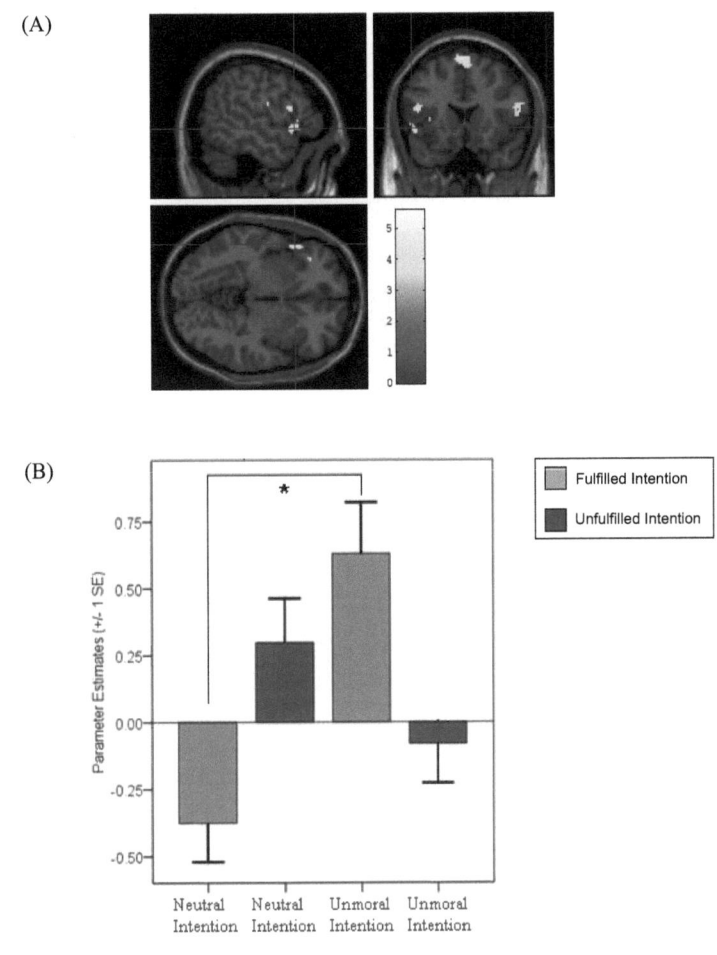

Fig. 7.6: (A) Functional changes in the amplitude of the HRF in the left ventrolateral prefrontal cortex (BA 47) associated with an intention by intention-outcome-relation interaction effect. (B) Post-hoc t-tests showed an activity increase for fulfilled immoral compared to fulfilled neutral intentions. BA, Brodmann's areas are approximate.

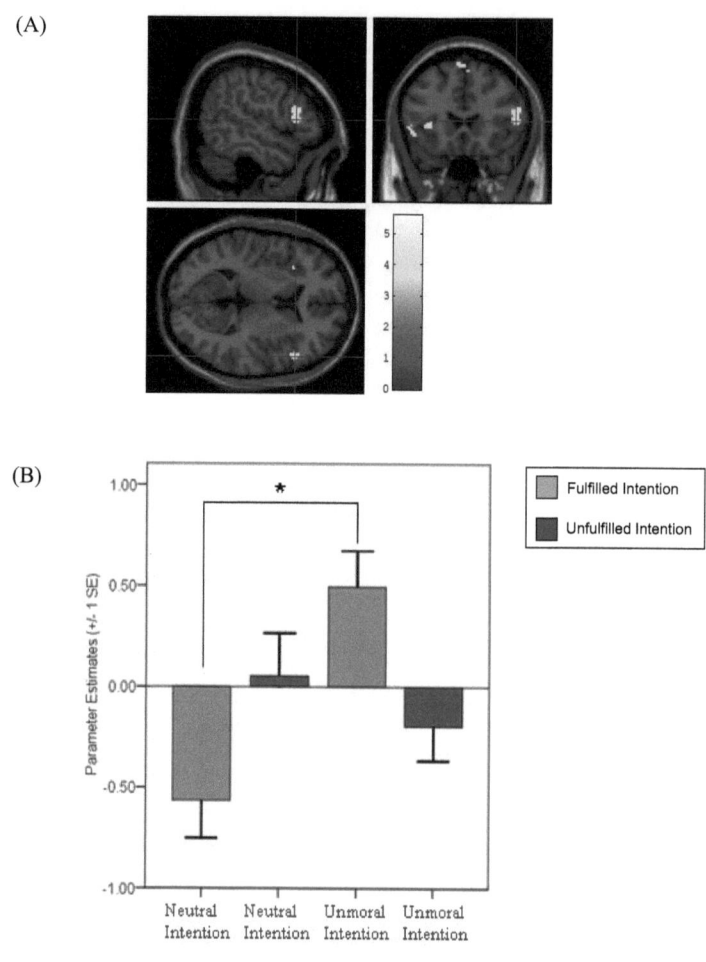

Fig. 7.7: (A) Functional changes in the amplitude of the HRF in the right ventrolateral prefrontal cortex (BA 45) associated with an intention by intention-outcome-relation interaction effect. (B) Post-hoc t-tests showed an activity increase for fulfilled immoral compared to fulfilled neutral intentions. Brodmann's areas are approximate.

8. DISCUSSION

STUDY II
EMOTIONS INFERRED FROM THE INTEGRATION OF IMMORAL INTENTIONS INTO INTENTION-OUTCOME-RELATIONS

This thesis investigated the neural network involved in intention-based emotion attribution. While the first study explored emotion attribution based on intention-outcome-relations, the second experiment aimed at investigating emotion attribution based on the integration of an actor's immoral intention into intention-outcome-relations. In the emotion attribution conditions a protagonist's neutral or immoral intention either matched or mismatched the outcome of the intended action. Further, a paralleled non-mental control condition was used. Chapter 8.1 discusses the behavioural findings, followed by the discussion of the functional findings (chapter 8.2) and a summary (chapter 8.3).

8.1 Behavioural findings

First, more negative emotions such as embarrassment and sadness were attributed in relation to immoral compared to neutral intentions, irrespective of the intention-outcome-relation. Second, the attribution of positive emotions varied with both the actor's intention and the intention-outcome-relation. That is, particularly in the case of fulfilled immoral intentions, an intermediate intensity of happiness, pride, and satisfaction was attributed. Moreover, the fulfilment of an immoral intention resulted in attributing the greatest intensity of the more immoral emotion schadenfreude. Therefore, specifically in the case of fulfilled immoral intentions, a mixture of different emotions was attributed: negative emotions and subdued positive emotions on the one hand, and the greatest amount of schadenfreude on the other hand. The results, therefore, may indicate that adults particularly attribute mixed emotions in cases where immoral intentions are fulfilled. This interpretation is supported by developmental findings which also observed the attribution of mixed emotions in relation to transgression scenarios during adulthood (Lagattuta, 2005).

Moreover, the results show that while the intensity of positive emotion attributions was a function of both other's immoral intentions and the intention-outcome-relation, the attribution of the negative emotions sadness and embarrassment was not affected by the interaction of theses factors. These findings suggest that, at least in adulthood, the intensity of positive, probably more goal-oriented emotions may be affected by the integration of immoral intentions into intention-outcome-relations. In contrast, the intensity of negative, probably more moral emotions seems to remain constant. This interpretation is supported by a developmental study which observed that during adolescence the intensity of the moral emotion guilt that was attributed to a victimizer remained stable irrespective of an onlooker's emotional reaction. In contrast, the intensity of positive emotions decreased with a disapproving onlooker compared to a mistakenly pleased onlooker (Murgatroyd & Robinson, 1997).

8.2 Neuroimaging findings

This study aimed at investigating the functional basis associated with emotions inferred from the integration of immoral intentions into the processing of intention-outcome-relations. As was expected, such interaction effects were found in the pre-SMA (BA 6) and the bilateral ventrolateral prefrontal cortex (VLPFC, BA 45/47). These brain regions showed an activity increase associated with emotions inferred from unfulfilled immoral intentions compared to fulfilled neutral intentions.

First, the pre-SMA activity increase associated with emotions inferred from fulfilled immoral intentions is supported by other studies showing that the pre-SMA is involved in the processing of intentional transgression (Berthoz et al., 2002; Finger et al., 2006). Further, in study one of this thesis, the pre-SMA activity was observed to be associated with emotions inferred from intention-outcome-relations. Based on this result, it was argued that even adults seem to infer others' emotions by matching their intention to the outcome situation rather than by processing it independent of reality cues (chapter 4.2.1). The present results extend the previous findings by suggesting that also immoral intentions, particularly fulfilled immoral intentions, may be processed in relation to situational cues rather than being processed independent of reality cues. Further, as argued in chapter 4.2.1, the pre-SMA plays an important role in the inhibition of automatic responses (Mostofsky & Simmonds, 2008). Therefore, for emotion attribution based on fulfilled immoral intentions, the pre-SMA activity increase indicates that participants may have suppressed an automatic intention-outcome-match response, which is probably based on a goal-oriented intention-outcome-matching strategy (e.g., feeling good = the intention to reach a goal matches the outcome). Instead, as indexed by the attribution of mixed emotions, participants may have given a more controlled intention-outcome-match response, which may have been based on simultaneously computing a goal-oriented and a morally-oriented intention-outcome-matching strategy (e.g., feeling mixed emotions = the intention to reach a goal matches a goal-oriented outcome + the intention not to harm mismatches a morally-oriented outcome).

This interpretation is further supported by the activity increase in the bilateral ventrolateral prefrontal cortex (BA 45 and BA 47) associated with emotion attribution based on fulfilled immoral intentions compared to fulfilled neutral intentions. As described before in chapter 4.2.3, while the anterior VLPFC (BA 47) is supposed to be involved in the controlled access to stored conceptual representations, the mid-VLPFC (BA 45) is argued to support a domain-general selection process that operates post-retrieval to resolve competition among active representations (Badre & Wagner, 2007). Therefore, the present findings suggest that the controlled intention-outcome-matching strategy that is assumed to underlie emotion attribution based on fulfilled immoral intentions may have been based on both script retrieval and on resolving a conflict between a more goal-oriented (e.g., 'people feel good when their intentions match the outcome') and a more morally-oriented script (e.g., 'people feel sad when they cause harm').

Interestingly and contrary to expectation, the present results revealed an activity increase in the pre-SMA for emotions inferred from fulfilled immoral intentions with no additional recruitment of brain regions implicated in representational operations, particularly the dorsal medial prefrontal cortex (DMPFC). This negative finding, however, is not consistent with other studies which observed, in addition to an increase in premotor activity, a DMPFC activity increase for emotions inferred from intentional versus unintentional transgression trials (Berthoz et al., 2002; Finger et al., 2006). The diverging findings could be due to differences with respect to an explicit versus implicit presentation of the protagonist's intention. While in the present study the actor's intention was explicitly stated, in previous studies the actor's intention was not explicitly presented, and therefore had to be indirectly inferred from the actor's behaviour. Therefore, the present results indicate that when intentions are explicitly stated, the integration of an actor's immoral intention into the processing of intention-outcome-relations may be solely based on intention-outcome-matching strategies without additionally processing other's immoral intentions independent of reality cues. In contrast, in cases where participants cannot simply rely on intention-outcome-matching strategies, the recruitment of those brain regions may be necessary that are involved in representational operations. This assumption is supported by a recent study on the neural network involved in the interaction between false belief reasoning and moral judgements in intention-outcome-scenarios (Young et al., 2007). In this study, the intention-outcome-relation was made explicit. Interestingly, while the rostral MPFC was found to be involved in attempted harm trials where the victimizer's behaviour was based on a false belief about reality, it was not involved in intended harm scenes where the victimizer did not hold a false belief about reality.

Contrary to study one, in study two the activity in the ventromedial prefrontal cortex did not vary with the experimental conditions. This negative finding is likely due to differences in the duration of the emotion attribution trials, on which the analysis focused (study 1: 6 sec, study 2: 3 sec). As argued in chapter 4.2.4, the VMPFC signal decrease associated with emotion attribution, which was observed in study one, was supposed to be associated with a disengagement from self-referential processes towards task-related processes. Because subjects in study two had only half the time to reason about others' emotions, this may have prevented them from engaging in self-referential processes, and, as a consequence, the ventromedial prefrontal cortex may not have been recruited.

8.3 Summary

The behavioural results confirm that adults attribute mixed emotions based on fulfilled immoral intentions. Furthermore, particularly the intensity of positive, probably goal-oriented emotions seems to be affected by the integration of immoral intentions into intention-outcome-matches. In contrast, the intensity of negative, probably more moral emotions seems to remain constant, irrespective of the fulfilment of an immoral intention. As was expected, similar information processes would be associated with emotion attribution based on simple intention-outcome-relations and emotion attribution based on the integration of immoral intentions into intention-outcome-relations. The pre-SMA activity suggests that even in situations where subjects have to infer mixed emotions based on fulfilled immoral intentions, they likely process the immoral intention in relation to the outcome situation rather than processing an actor's immoral intention independent of reality cues. That is, particularly in the case of attributing mixed emotions inferred from fulfilled immoral intentions participants may have given a more controlled intention-outcome-match response which may have been based on simultaneously computing a goal-oriented and a morally-oriented intention-outcome-matching strategy. This intention-outcome-matching strategy, however, seems to be restricted to cases where other's intentions are explicitly stated, as indexed by the negative finding with respect to DMPFC recruitment. Further, it was argued that the intention-outcome-matching strategy, which is assumed to rely predominately on pre-SMA activity, may also be based on script retrieval, as indexed by the anterior VLPFC activity (BA 47). In addition, particularly for the processing of mixed emotions inferred from fulfilled immoral intentions, a conflict between a more goal-oriented and a more morally-oriented script may have been resolved post-retrieval, as indexed by the mid-VLPFC activity (BA 45).

9. GENERAL DISCUSSION AND PERSPECTIVES

The ability to infer another person's emotions from his or her intention is shortly acquired around the ability to understand false beliefs, the key ToM ability. False belief understanding is supposed to be an indicator of representational understanding. This thesis was the first extending research on the neural network involved in Theory of Mind (ToM) to intention-based emotion attribution. Based on developmental and neuronal findings, it was assumed that emotions inferred from intention-outcome-relations would be less associated with brain regions implicated in representational operations, particularly the dorsal medial prefrontal cortex (DMPFC) and the temporo-parietal-junction (TPJ). In contrast, specifically emotions inferred from fulfilled immoral intentions were assumed to be associated with brain regions involved in representational operations, specifically the DMPFC. Two experiments were conducted. Experiment 1 investigated emotion attribution based on intention-outcome-relations, an ability which precedes the ability to understand false beliefs. Experiment 2 was concerned with emotion attribution based on the integration of immoral intentions into intention-outcome-relations, an ability which develops shortly after false belief understanding.

First, neither the DMPFC nor the TPJ were observed to be involved in intention-based emotion attribution. This finding indicates that adults may attribute emotions, even mixed emotions in the case of fulfilled immoral intentions, without representational operations. Moreover, a similar neural network was observed when emotions were inferred from intention-outcome-relations and when emotions were inferred by integrating immoral intentions into intention-outcome-relations. This network particularly comprised the medial pre-supplementary motor area (pre-SMA, BA 6) and the ventrolateral prefrontal cortex (VLPFC, BA 45/47). This network was specifically active during emotion attribution based on unfulfilled intentions and on fulfilled immoral intentions. Regarding the pre-SMA activity, intention-based emotion attribution may be associated with a controlled intention-outcome-matching strategy. That is, at least in adulthood, emotions may be inferred by a controlled matching of an intention to an outcome situation, rather than by processing the intention independent of reality cues. More specifically, in the case of unfulfilled intentions, participants may have suppressed an automatic intention-outcome-matching response based on an expected intention-outcome-match situation. Instead, subjects may have adjusted the automatic intention-outcome-matching response to an unexpected intention-outcome-mismatch situation. Moreover, in the case of attributing mixed emotions inferred from fulfilled immoral intentions, participants may have simultaneously computed a goal-oriented and a morally-oriented intention-outcome-matching strategy. The assumption of a controlled intention-outcome-matching strategy in cases where either an intention mismatches an outcome situation, or where an immoral intention induces a mismatch between a goal-oriented and a morally-oriented intention-outcome-matching response, is further supported by anterior and mid-VLPFC activity. The VLPFC activity suggests that particularly for negative emotions inferred from unfulfilled intentions and for mixed emotions inferred from fulfilled immoral intentions, it may have been necessary to retrieve scripts in a controlled information processing modus, as indexed by the anterior VLPFC activity (BA 47). Moreover, specifically for the processing of mixed emotions inferred from fulfilled immoral intentions, adults may have resolved a conflict between a more goal-oriented and a more morally-oriented script, as indexed by the mid-VLPFC activity (BA 45).

In sum, the functional findings on emotions inferred from intention-outcome-relations indicate that even adult participants may have matched an actor's intention to an outcome situation rather than processing its intention, even its unfulfilled intention independent of reality cues. Therefore, intention-based emotion attribution, at least for neutral intentions, does not seem to require representational operations. Further, the functional findings on emotion attribution based on the integration of an immoral intention into intention-outcome-relations challenge developmental findings. Developmental evidence indicates that young children's happy victimizer responses based on fulfilled immoral intentions are a function of an immature representational understanding. The neuronal adult data speak against the assumption of representational operations underlying emotion attribution for immoral intentions. Instead, at least in adults, the neuronal findings suggest that the processing of mixed emotions inferred from fulfilled immoral intentions may be a function of an increasing ability to simultaneously compute diverging intention-outcome-matching strategies and to simultaneously process diverging intention-based emotion attribution scripts, rather than being a function of representational operations. To further test this assumption, a developmental study should investigate the brain regions associated with intention-based emotion attribution. Further, subsequent research should combine research on false belief understanding and intention-based emotion attribution by exploring the neural network involved in belief-based emotion attribution compared to intention-based emotion attribution.

10. SUMMARY

This thesis extends research on the neural network involved in Theory of Mind (ToM) to intention-based emotion attribution. Children acquire this ability around the ability to understand false beliefs. False belief understanding is the key ToM ability because of indicating representational understanding. Two experiments were conducted. In both experiments cartoon stories with verbal vignettes were presented. The experimental conditions only differed in their verbal vignettes. In experiment 1 fifteen healthy adults reasoned about emotions inferred from intention-outcome-relations, an ability which develops shortly before the acquirement of false belief understanding. In experiment 2 eighteen healthy adults attributed emotions based on integrating an actor's immoral intention into intention-outcome-relations, an ability that develops shortly after the development of false belief understanding. Based on developmental and neuronal findings, it was assumed that emotions inferred from intention-outcome-relations would be less associated with brain regions implicated in representational operations, in particular the dorsal medial prefrontal cortex (DMPFC) and the temporo-parietal-junction (TPJ). In contrast, specifically emotions inferred from fulfilled immoral intentions were assumed to be associated with brain regions involved in representational operations, specifically the DMPFC. In Experiment 1 the emotion attribution conditions varied depending on an actor's intention either matching or mismatching an outcome situation. In Experiment 2, in addition to the factor intention-outcome-relation, an actor either held a neutral or immoral intention (factor intention). In the emotion attribution picture following the story pictures, which depict an actor's intention and an outcome situation, subjects had to reason about the actor's emotion based on its intention and the outcome of the intended action. The fMRI analysis focused on the functional activity associated with the emotion attribution cue. The emotion attribution picture was followed by a response picture presenting different emotion dimensions (Experiment 1: neutral, positive, negative; Experiment 2: positive, negative). Besides the emotion attribution conditions, a non-mental reality judgement condition was used. Following the fMRI session, a rating task with different emotion dimensions was conducted to get more specific emotion attribution results. Neither the DMPFC nor the TPJ was involved in intention-based emotion attribution. Instead, a neuronal network specifically comprising the pre-supplementary motor area (pre-SMA) and the ventrolateral prefrontal cortex (VLPFC) was associated with negative emotions inferred from unfulfilled intentions (experiment 1) and with mixed emotions inferred from fulfilled immoral intentions (experiment 2). These findings indicate that intention-based emotion attribution, including the processing of mixed emotions inferred from fulfilled immoral intentions, may be a function of an increasing ability to simultaneously compute diverging intention-outcome-matching strategies and to simultaneously process diverging intention-based emotion attribution scripts, rather than being a function of representational operations.

11. REFERENCES

Abell, F., Happe, F., & Frith, U. (2000). Do triangles play tricks? Attribution of mental states to animated shapes in normal and abnormal development. *Cogn Emot, 15*, 1-16.

Aichhorn, M., Perner, J., Weiss, B., Kronbichler, M., Staffen, W., & Ladurner, G. (2008a). Temporo-parietal Junction Activity in Theory-of-Mind Tasks: Falseness, Beliefs, or Attention. *J Cogn Neurosci..*

Aichhorn, M., Perner, J., Weiss, B., Kronbichler, M., Staffen, W., & Ladurner, G. (2008b). Temporo-parietal Junction Activity in Theory-of-Mind Tasks: Falseness, Beliefs, or Attention. *J Cogn Neurosci..*

Aichhorn, M., Perner, J., Weiss, B., Kronbichler, M., Staffen, W., & Ladurner, G. (2008c). Temporo-parietal Junction Activity in Theory-of-Mind Tasks: Falseness, Beliefs, or Attention. *J Cogn Neurosci..*

Aichhorn, M., Perner, J., Weiss, B., Kronbichler, M., Staffen, W., & Ladurner, G. (2008d). Temporo-parietal Junction Activity in Theory-of-Mind Tasks: Falseness, Beliefs, or Attention. *J Cogn Neurosci..*

Aichhorn, M., Perner, J., Weiss, B., Kronbichler, M., Staffen, W., & Ladurner, G. (2008e). Temporo-parietal Junction Activity in Theory-of-Mind Tasks: Falseness, Beliefs, or Attention. *J Cogn Neurosci..*

Aichhorn, M., Perner, J., Weiss, B., Kronbichler, M., Staffen, W., & Ladurner, G. (2008f). Temporo-parietal Junction Activity in Theory-of-Mind Tasks: Falseness, Beliefs, or Attention. *J Cogn Neurosci..*

Amodio, D. M. & Frith, C. D. (2006). Meeting of minds: the medial frontal cortex and social cognition. *Nat.Rev.Neurosci., 7*, 268-277.

Arsenio, W. F., Gold, J., & Adams, E. (2006). Children's conceptions and displays of moral emotions. In M.Killen & J. G. Smetana (Eds.), *Handbook of moral development* (pp. 581-609). Mahwah, New Jersey: Lawrence Erlbaum.

Arsenio, W. F. & Kramer, R. (1992). Victimizers and their victims: children's conceptions of the mixed emotional consequences of moral transgressions. *Child Dev., 63*, 915-927.

Arsenio, W. F. & Lover, A. (1995). Children's conceptions of sociomoral affect: Happy victimizers, mixed emotions, and other expectancies. In M.Killen & D. Hart (Eds.), *Morality in everyday life: Developmental perspectives* (pp. 87-128). Cambridge: Cambridge University Press.

Astington, J. W. (1993). *The child's discovery of the mind.* Cambridge, Mass: Harvard University Press.

Astington, J. W. (1999a). The language of intention. Three ways of doing it. In P.D.Zelazo, J. W. Astington, & D. R. Olson (Eds.), *Developing theories of intention: Social understanding and self-control* (pp. 295-315). Mahwah, NJ: Lawrence Erlbaum Associates.

Astington, J. W. (2001b). The paradox of intention: Assessing children's metarepresentational understanding. In L.J.Malle, L. J. Moses, & D. A. Baldwin (Eds.), *Intentions and intentionality: Foundations of social cognition* (pp. 85-103). Cambridge, MA: MIT Press.

Astington, J. W. (2004). Bridging the gap between Theory of Mind and moral reasoning. *New directions for child and adolescent development, 103*, 63-83.

Badre, D. (2008). Cognitive control, hierarchy, and the rostro-caudal organization of the frontal lobes. *Trends Cogn Sci., 12*, 193-200.

Badre, D. & D'Esposito, M. (2007). Functional magnetic resonance imaging evidence for a hierarchical organization of the prefrontal cortex. *J Cogn Neurosci., 19*, 2082-2099.

Badre, D. & Wagner, A. D. (2007). Left ventrolateral prefrontal cortex and the cognitive control of memory. *Neuropsychologia, 45*, 2883-2901.

Baird, J. A. & Astington, J. W. (2004). The role of mental state understanding in the development of moral cognition and moral action. *New directions for child and adolescent development, 103*, 37-49.

Baird, J. A. & Astington, J. W. (2005). The development of the intention concept: From the observable world to the unobservable mind. In R.R.Hassin, J. S. Uleman, & J. Bargh (Eds.), *The new unconscious* (pp. 256-276). Oxford: Oxford University Press.

Baird, J. A. & Moses, L. J. (2002). Do preschoolers appreciate that identical actions may be motivated by different intentions. *Journal of cognition and development, 2*, 413-448.

Barden, R. C., Zelko, F. A., Duncan, S. W., & Masters, J. C. (1980). Children's consensual knowledge about the experiential determinants of emotion. *J Pers.Soc.Psychol., 39*, 968-976.

Baron-Cohen, S., Leslie, A. M., & Frith, U. (1985). Does the autistic child have a "theory of mind"? *Cognition, 21*, 37-46.

Baron-Cohen, S., Leslie, A. M., & Frith, U. (1986). Mechanical, behavioural and intentional understanding of pictures in autistic children. *Br.J.Dev Psychol., 4*, 113-125.

Baron-Cohen, S., Ring, H. A., Wheelwright, S., Bullmore, E. T., Brammer, M. J., Simmons, A. et al. (1999). Social intelligence in the normal and autistic brain: an fMRI study. *Eur.J Neurosci, 11*, 1891-1898.

Beer, J. S. (2007). The default self: feeling good or being right? *Trends Cogn Sci., 11*, 187-189.

Berthoz, S., Armony, J. L., Blair, R. J., & Dolan, R. J. (2002). An fMRI study of intentional and unintentional (embarrassing) violations of social norms. *Brain, 125*, 1696-1708.

Brunet, E., Sarfati, Y., Hardy-Bayle, M. C., & Decety, J. (2000). A PET investigation of the attribution of intentions with a nonverbal task. *Neuroimage, 11*, 157-166.

Buccino, G., Baumgaertner, A., Colle, L., Buechel, C., Rizzolatti, G., & Binkofski, F. (2007). The neural basis for understanding non-intended actions. *Neuroimage, 36 Suppl 2*, T119-T127.

Buckner, R. L., Andrews-Hanna, J. R., & Schacter, D. L. (2008). The brain's default network: anatomy, function, and relevance to disease. *Ann.N.Y.Acad.Sci., 1124*, 1-38.

Buckner, R. L. & Carroll, D. C. (2007). Self-projection and the brain. *Trends Cogn Sci., 11*, 49-57.

Castelli, F., Frith, C., Happe, F., & Frith, U. (2002). Autism, Asperger syndrome and brain mechanisms for the attribution of mental states to animated shapes. *Brain, 125*, 1839-1849.

Castelli, F., Happe, F., Frith, U., & Frith, C. (2000). Movement and mind: a functional imaging study of perception and interpretation of complex intentional movement patterns. *Neuroimage, 12*, 314-325.

Collins, D. L., Neelin, P., Peters, T. M., & Evans, A. C. (1994). Automatic 3D intersubject registration of MR volumetric data in standardized Talairach space. *J.Comput.Assist.Tomogr., 18*, 192-205.

Corbetta, M., Patel, G., & Shulman, G. L. (2008). The reorienting system of the human brain: from environment to theory of mind. *Neuron, 58*, 306-324.

Feinfield, K. A., Lee, P. P., Flavell, E. R., Green, F. L., & Flavell, J. H. (1999). Young children's understanding of intention. *Cognitive Development, 14*, 463-468.

Finger, E. C., Marsh, A. A., Kamel, N., Mitchell, D. G., & Blair, J. R. (2006). Caught in the act: the impact of audience on the neural response to morally and socially inappropriate behavior. *Neuroimage., 33*, 414-421.

Fletcher, P. C., Happe, F., Frith, U., Baker, S. C., Dolan, R. J., Frackowiak, R. S. et al. (1995). Other minds in the brain: a functional imaging study of "theory of mind" in story comprehension. *Cognition, 57*, 109-128.

Friston, K. J., Fletcher, P., Josephs, O., Holmes, A., Rugg, M. D., & Turner, R. (1998). Event-related fMRI: characterizing differential responses. *Neuroimage, 7*, 30-40.

Friston, K. J., Penny, W., Phillips, C., Kiebel, S., Hinton, G., & Ashburner, J. (2002). Classical and Bayesian inference in neuroimaging: theory. *Neuroimage, 16*, 465-483.

Friston, K. J., Rotshtein, P., Geng, J. J., Sterzer, P., & Henson, R. N. (2006). A critique of functional localisers. *Neuroimage., 30*, 1077-1087.

Frith, C. D. & Frith, U. (1999). Interacting minds--a biological basis. *Science, 286*, 1692-1695.

Frith, C. D. & Frith, U. (2006). The neural basis of mentalizing. *Neuron, 50*, 531-534.

Frith, U. & Frith, C. D. (2003). Development and neurophysiology of mentalizing. *Philos.Trans.R.Soc.Lond B Biol.Sci., 358*, 459-473.

Gallagher, H. L. & Frith, C. D. (2003). Functional imaging of 'theory of mind'. *Trends Cogn.Sci., 7*, 77-83.

Gallagher, H. L., Happe, F., Brunswick, N., Fletcher, P. C., Frith, U., & Frith, C. D. (2000). Reading the mind in cartoons and stories: an fMRI study of 'theory of mind' in verbal and nonverbal tasks. *Neuropsychologia, 38*, 11-21.

Gallese, V. (2007). Before and below 'theory of mind': embodied simulation and the neural correlates of social cognition. *Philos.Trans.R.Soc.Lond B Biol.Sci., 362*, 659-669.

Gallese, V., Cossu, G., & Sinigaglia, C. (2009). Motor cognition and its role in the phylogeny and ontogeny of action understanding. *Dev.Psychol., 45*, 103-113.

Gobbini, M. I., Koralek, A. C., Bryan, R. E., Montgomery, K. J., & Haxby, J. V. (2007). Two Takes on the Social Brain: A Comparison of Theory of Mind Tasks. *J.Cogn Neurosci., 19*, 1803-1814.

Greene, J. & Haidt, J. (2002). How (and where) does moral judgment work? *Trends Cogn Sci., 6*, 517-523.

Greene, J. D., Sommerville, R. B., Nystrom, L. E., Darley, J. M., & Cohen, J. D. (2001). An fMRI investigation of emotional engagement in moral judgment. *Science, 293*, 2105-2108.

Gusnard, D. A., Akbudak, E., Shulman, G. L., & Raichle, M. E. (2001). Medial prefrontal cortex and self-referential mental activity: relation to a default mode of brain function. *Proc.Natl.Acad.Sci.U.S.A, 98*, 4259-4264.

Gusnard, D. A., Raichle, M. E., & Raichle, M. E. (2001). Searching for a baseline: functional imaging and the resting human brain. *Nat.Rev.Neurosci., 2*, 685-694.

Hadwin, J. & Perner, J. (1991). Pleased and surprised: Children's cognitive theory of emotion. *Br.J.Dev Psychol., 9*, 215-234.

Hassabis, D. & Maguire, E. A. (2007). Deconstructing episodic memory with construction. *Trends Cogn Sci., 11*, 299-306.

Heberlein, A. S., Adolphs, R., Tranel, D., & Damasio, H. (2004). Cortical regions for judgments of emotions and personality traits from point-light walkers. *J Cogn Neurosci, 16*, 1143-1158.

Heberlein, A. S. & Saxe, R. R. (2005). Dissociation between emotion and personality judgments: convergent evidence from functional neuroimaging. *Neuroimage, 28*, 770-777.

Heekeren, H. R., Wartenburger, I., Schmidt, H., Schwintowski, H. P., & Villringer, A. (2003). An fMRI study of simple ethical decision-making. *Neuroreport, 14*, 1215-1219.

Henson, R. N. A. & Penny, W. D. (2003). *ANOVAs and SPM*. Wellcome Department of Imaging Neuroscience.

Hill, E. L. & Frith, U. (2003). Understanding autism: insights from mind and brain. *Philos.Trans.R.Soc.Lond B Biol.Sci., 358*, 281-289.

Hynes, C. A., Baird, A. A., & Grafton, S. T. (2006). Differential role of the orbital frontal lobe in emotional versus cognitive perspective-taking. *Neuropsychologia, 44*, 374-383.

Iacoboni, M. (2008). Imitation, Empathy, and Mirror Neurons. *Annu.Rev.Psychol, 60*, 653-670.

Iacoboni, M. & Dapretto, M. (2006). The mirror neuron system and the consequences of its dysfunction. *Nat.Rev.Neurosci., 7*, 942-951.

Iacoboni, M. & Mazziotta, J. C. (2007). Mirror neuron system: basic findings and clinical applications. *Ann.Neurol., 62*, 213-218.

Iacoboni, M., Molnar-Szakacs, I., Gallese, V., Buccino, G., Mazziotta, J. C., & Rizzolatti, G. (2005). Grasping the intentions of others with one's own mirror neuron system. *PLoS.Biol., 3*, 529-535.

Kedia, G., Berthoz, S., Wessa, M., Hilton, D., & Martinot, J. L. (2008). An agent harms a victim: a functional magnetic resonance imaging study on specific moral emotions. *J Cogn Neurosci., 20*, 1788-1798.

Keller, M., Gummerum, M., Wang, X. T., & Lindsey, S. (2004). Understanding perspectives and emotions in contract violation: development of deontic and moral reasoning. *Child Dev, 75*, 614-635.

Keller, M., Lourenco, O., Malti, T., & Saalbach, H. (2003). The multifaceted phenomenom of 'happy victimizer': a cross-cultural comparison of moral emotions. *Br.J.Dev Psychol., 21*, 1-18.

Knutson, B., Taylor, J., Kaufman, M., Peterson, R., & Glover, G. (2005). Distributed neural representation of expected value. *J.Neurosci., 25*, 4806-4812.

Koechlin, E. & Summerfield, C. (2007). An information theoretical approach to prefrontal executive function. *Trends Cogn Sci., 11*, 229-235.

Krettenauer, T. & Eichler, D. (2006). Adolescents' self-attributed moral emotions following a moral transgression: Relations with delinquency, confidence in moral judgment and age. *Br.J.Dev Psychol., 24*, 489-506.

Lagattuta, K. (2005). When you shouldn't do what you want to do: Young children's understanding of desires, rules, and emotions. *Child Dev., 76*, 713-733.

Lalonde, C. E. & Chandler, M. J. (2002). Children's understanding of interpretation. *New Ideas in Psychology, 20*, 163-198.

Lau, H. C., Rogers, R. D., Haggard, P., & Passingham, R. E. (2004). Attention to intention. *Science, 303*, 1208-1210.

Libet, B., Gleason, C. A., Wright, E. W., & Pearl, D. K. (1983). Time of conscious intention to act in relation to onset of cerebral activity (readiness-potential). The unconscious initiation of a freely voluntary act. *Brain, 106*, 623-642.

Lieberman, M. D. (2007). Social cognitive neuroscience: a review of core processes. *Annu.Rev.Psychol., 58*, 259-289.

Lourenco, O. (1997). Children's attributions of moral emotions to victimizers: Some data, doubts and suggestions. *Br.J.Dev Psychol., 15*, 425-438.

Martin, A. & Weisberg, J. (2003). Neural Foundations For Understanding Social And Mechanical Concepts. *Cogn Neuropsychol., 20*, 575-587.

McKiernan, K. A., D'Angelo, B. R., Kaufman, J. N., & Binder, J. R. (2006). Interrupting the "stream of consciousness": An fMRI investigation. *Neuroimage., 29*, 1185-1191.

Mitchell, J. P. (2006). Mentalizing and Marr: an information processing approach to the study of social cognition. *Brain Res., 1079*, 66-75.

Moll, J., Oliveira-Souza, R., Bramati, I. E., & Grafman, J. (2002). Functional networks in emotional moral and nonmoral social judgments. *Neuroimage., 16*, 696-703.

Moll, J., Oliveira-Souza, R., Eslinger, P. J., Bramati, I. E., Mourao-Miranda, J., Andreiuolo, P. A. et al. (2002). The neural correlates of moral sensitivity: a functional magnetic resonance imaging investigation of basic and moral emotions. *J Neurosci., 22*, 2730-2736.

Montgomery, D. E. & Montgomery, D. A. (1999). The influence of movement and outcome on young children's attributions of intention. *Br.J.Dev Psychol., 17*, 245-261.

Mostofsky, S. H. & Simmonds, D. J. (2008). Response inhibition and response selection: two sides of the same coin. *J Cogn Neurosci., 20,* 751-761.

Murgatroyd, S. J. & Robinson, E. J. (1993). Children's judgment of emotion following moral transgression. *Int.J Behav Dev., 16,* 93-111.

Murgatroyd, S. J. & Robinson, E. J. (1997). Children's and Adults' Attributions of Emotion to a Wrongdoer: The Influence of the Onlooker's Reaction. *Cogn Emot, 11,* 83-101.

Nakamura, K., Kawashima, R., Ito, K., Sugiura, M., Kato, T., Nakamura, A. et al. (1999). Activation of the right inferior frontal cortex during assessment of facial emotion. *J Neurophysiol., 82,* 1610-1614.

Northoff, G. & Bermpohl, F. (2004). Cortical midline structures and the self. *Trends Cogn Sci., 8,* 102-107.

Nunner-Winkler, G. & Sodian, B. (1988). Children's understanding of moral emotions. *Child Dev., 59,* 1323-1338.

Ochsner, K. N., Hughes, B., Robertson, E. R., Cooper, J. C., & Gabrieli, J. D. (2008). Neural Systems Supporting the Control of Affective and Cognitive Conflicts. *J Cogn Neurosci.*.

Ochsner, K. N., Knierim, K., Ludlow, D. H., Hanelin, J., Ramachandran, T., Glover, G. et al. (2004). Reflecting upon feelings: an fMRI study of neural systems supporting the attribution of emotion to self and other. *J.Cogn Neurosci., 16,* 1746-1772.

Olsson, A. & Ochsner, K. N. (2008). The role of social cognition in emotion. *Trends Cogn Sci., 12,* 65-71.

Owen, A. M., McMillan, K. M., Laird, A. R., & Bullmore, E. (2005). N-back working memory paradigm: a meta-analysis of normative functional neuroimaging studies. *Hum.Brain Mapp., 25,* 46-59.

Perner, J. (1991a). On representing that: The assymetry between belief and desire in children's theory of mind. In D.Frye & C. Moore (Eds.), *Children's theories of mind: Mental states and social understanding* (pp. 139-155). Hillsdale, New Jersey: Lawrence Erlbaum.

Perner, J. (1991b). *Understanding the representational mind.* Cambridge, Massachusetts: MIT Press.

Perner, J. & Aichhorn, M. (2008). Theory of mind, language and the temporoparietal junction mystery. *Trends Cogn Sci., 12,* 123-126.

Perner, J., Aichhorn, M., Kronbichler, M., Staffen, W., & Ladurner, G. (2006). Thinking of mental and other representations: the roles of left and right temporo-parietal junction. *Soc Neurosci., 1,* 245-258.

Perner, J. & Leekam, S. (2008). The curious incident of the photo that was accused of being false: issues of domain specificity in development, autism, and brain imaging. *Q.J.Exp.Psychol.(Colchester.), 61,* 76-89.

Petrides, M. (2005). Lateral prefrontal cortex: architectonic and functional organization. *Philos.Trans.R.Soc Lond B Biol.Sci., 360,* 781-795.

Raichle, M. E., MacLeod, A. M., Snyder, A. Z., Powers, W. J., Gusnard, D. A., & Shulman, G. L. (2001). A default mode of brain function. *Proc.Natl.Acad.Sci.U.S.A, 98*, 676-682.

Ramnani, N. & Owen, A. M. (2004). Anterior prefrontal cortex: insights into function from anatomy and neuroimaging. *Nat.Rev.Neurosci., 5*, 184-194.

Rizzolatti, G. & Fabbri-Destro, M. (2008). The mirror system and its role in social cognition. *Curr.Opin.Neurobiol., 18*, 179-184.

Rizzolatti, G. & Sinigaglia, C. (2007). Mirror neurons and motor intentionality. *Funct.Neurol., 22*, 205-210.

Ruby, P. & Decety, J. (2004). How would you feel versus how do you think she would feel? A neuroimaging study of perspective-taking with social emotions. *J.Cogn Neurosci., 16*, 988-999.

Rushworth, M. F., Behrens, T. E., Rudebeck, P. H., & Walton, M. E. (2007). Contrasting roles for cingulate and orbitofrontal cortex in decisions and social behaviour. *Trends Cogn Sci., 11*, 168-176.

Saxe, R. (2006). Uniquely human social cognition. *Curr.Opin.Neurobiol., 16*, 235-239.

Saxe, R. & Baron-Cohen, S. (2006). The neuroscience of theory of mind. *Soc Neurosci., 1*, i-ix.

Saxe, R., Carey, S., & Kanwisher, N. (2004). Understanding other minds: linking developmental psychology and functional neuroimaging. *Annu.Rev.Psychol., 55*, 87-124.

Saxe, R. & Kanwisher, N. (2003). People thinking about thinking people. The role of the temporo-parietal junction in "theory of mind". *Neuroimage, 19*, 1835-1842.

Saxe, R. & Powell, L. J. (2006). It's the thought that counts: specific brain regions for one component of theory of mind. *Psychol Sci., 17*, 692-699.

Saxe, R., Schulz, L. E., & Jiang, Y. V. (2006). Reading minds versus following rules: dissociating theory of mind and executive control in the brain. *Soc Neurosci., 1*, 284-298.

Saxe, R. & Wexler, A. (2005). Making sense of another mind: The role of the right temporo-parietal junction. *Neuropsychologia, 43*, 1391-1399.

Schaich, B. J., Hynes, C., Van, H. J., Grafton, S., & Sinnott-Armstrong, W. (2006). Consequences, action, and intention as factors in moral judgments: an FMRI investigation. *J.Cogn Neurosci., 18*, 803-817.

Schult, C. A. (2002). Children's understanding of the distinction between intentions and desires. *Child Dev, 73*, 1727-1747.

Schulte-Ruther, M., Markowitsch, H. J., Fink, G. R., & Piefke, M. (2007). Mirror neuron and theory of mind mechanisms involved in face-to-face interactions: a functional magnetic resonance imaging approach to empathy. *J.Cogn Neurosci., 19*, 1354-1372.

Schultz, R. T. (2005). Developmental deficits in social perception in autism: the role of the amygdala and fusiform face area. *Int.J Dev.Neurosci., 23*, 125-141.

Schultz, R. T., Grelotti, D. J., Klin, A., Kleinman, J., Van der, G. C., Marois, R. et al. (2003). The role of the fusiform face area in social cognition: implications for the pathobiology of autism. *Philos.Trans.R.Soc.Lond B Biol.Sci., 358*, 415-427.

Searle, J. R. (1983). *Intentionality: An essay in the philosophy of mind*. Cambridge, England: Cambridge University Press.

Shin, L. M., Dougherty, D. D., Orr, S. P., Pitman, R. K., Lasko, M., Macklin, M. L. et al. (2000). Activation of anterior paralimbic structures during guilt-related script-driven imagery. *Biol.Psychiatry, 48*, 43-50.

Sodian, B. (2005). Tiefgreifende Entwicklungsstörung. Autismus. In P.F.Schlottke, R. K. Silbereisen, S. Scheider, & G. W. Lauth (Eds.), *Enzyklopädie der Psychologie. Serie II: Klinische Psychologie. Bd. 6: Störungen des Kindes- und Jugendalters* (pp. 419-452). Göttingen: Hogrefe.

Sodian, B. & Thoermer, C. (2006). Theory of Mind. In W.Schneider & B. Sodian (Eds.), *Enzyklopädie der Psychologie, Serie V: Entwicklung, Band 2: Kognitive Entwicklung* (pp. 495-608). Göttingen: Hogrefe.

Sokol, B. (2004). *Children's conceptions of agency and morality: Making sense of the happy victimizer phenomenon*. The University of British Columbia.

Sokol, B. & Chandler, M. J. (2004). The relation between children's developing theories of mind and the happy victimizer phenomenom. In Ghent, Belgium.

Sokol, B., Chandler, M. J., & Jones, C. (2004). From mechanical to autonomous agency: the relationship between children's moral judgments and their developing theories of mind. *New directions for child and adolescent development, 103*, 19-36.

Sommer, M., Döhnel, K., Meinhardt, J., & Hajak, G. (2008). Decoding of affective facial expressions in the context of emotional situations. *Neuropsychologia, 46*, 2615-2621.

Sommer, M., Döhnel, K., Sodian, B., Meinhardt, J., Thoermer, C., & Hajak, G. (2007). Neural correlates of true and false belief reasoning. *Neuroimage, 35*, 1378-1384.

Steele, J. D. & Lawrie, S. M. (2004). Segregation of cognitive and emotional function in the prefrontal cortex: a stereotactic meta-analysis. *Neuroimage., 21*, 868-875.

Stein, N. L. & Levine, L. J. (1989). The causal organisation of emotional knowledge. *Cogn Emot, 3*, 343-378.

Stone, V. E. & Gerrans, P. (2006). What's domain-specific about theory of mind? *Soc Neurosci., 1*, 309-319.

Takahashi, H., Yahata, N., Koeda, M., Matsuda, T., Asai, K., & Okubo, Y. (2004). Brain activation associated with evaluative processes of guilt and embarrassment: an fMRI study. *Neuroimage., 23*, 967-974.

Tanaka, S., Honda, M., & Sadato, N. (2005). Modality-specific cognitive function of medial and lateral human Brodmann area 6. *J.Neurosci., 25*, 496-501.

Tavares, P., Lawrence, A. D., & Barnard, P. J. (2008). Paying attention to social meaning: an FMRI study. *Cereb.Cortex, 18*, 1876-1885.

Vanderwal, T., Hunyadi, E., Grupe, D. W., Connors, C. M., & Schultz, R. T. (2008). Self, mother and abstract other: an fMRI study of reflective social processing. *Neuroimage., 41*, 1437-1446.

Wager, T. D. & Smith, E. E. (2003). Neuroimaging studies of working memory: a meta-analysis. *Cogn Affect.Behav.Neurosci., 3*, 255-274.

Walter, H., Adenzato, M., Ciaramidaro, A., Enrici, I., Pia, L., & Bara, B. G. (2004). Understanding intentions in social interaction: the role of the anterior paracingulate cortex. *J Cogn Neurosci, 16*, 1854-1863.

Walton, M. E., Devlin, J. T., & Rushworth, M. F. (2004). Interactions between decision making and performance monitoring within prefrontal cortex. *Nat.Neurosci., 7*, 1259-1265.

Wellman, H. M. (1990). *The child's theory of mind*. Cambridge, Massachusetts: MIT Press.

Wellman, H. M. & Banerjee, M. (1991). Mind and emotion: Children's understanding of the emotional consequences of beliefs and desires. *Br.J.Dev Psychol., 9*, 191-214.

Wellman, H. M., Cross, D., & Watson, J. (2001). Meta-analysis of theory-of-mind development: the truth about false belief. *Child Dev., 72*, 655-684.

Wellman, H. M. & Woolley, J. D. (1990). From simple desires to ordinary beliefs: the early development of everyday psychology. *Cognition, 35*, 245-275.

Wicker, B., Perrett, D. I., Baron-Cohen, S., & Decety, J. (2003). Being the target of another's emotion: a PET study. *Neuropsychologia, 41*, 139-146.

Wiersma, N. & Laupa, M. (2000). Young children's conceptions of the emotional consequences of varied social events. *Merill-Palmer Quarterly, 46*, 325-341.

Wimmer, H. & Perner, J. (1983). Beliefs about beliefs: representation and constraining function of wrong beliefs in young children's understanding of deception. *Cognition, 13*, 103-128.

Young, L., Cushman, F., Hauser, M., & Saxe, R. (2007). The neural basis of the interaction between theory of mind and moral judgment. *Proc.Natl.Acad.Sci.U.S.A, 104*, 8235-8240.

Young, L. & Saxe, R. (2008). The neural basis of belief encoding and integration in moral judgment. *Neuroimage., 40*, 1912-1920.

Yuill, N. (1984). Young children's coordination of motive and outcome in judgements of satisfaction and morality. *Br.J.Dev Psychol., 2*, 73-81.

Yuill, N., Perner, J., Pearson, A., Peerbhoy, D., & van den Ende, J. (1996). Children's changing understanding of wicked desires: From objective to subjective and moral. *Br.J.Dev Psychol., 14*, 457-475.

APPENDIX A

INDEX OF FIGURES AND TABLES

Index of Figures

Fig. 1.1: Involvement of the medial prefrontal cortex in ToM. More rostral parts of the medial prefrontal cortex (MPFC) are associated with false belief reasoning (red), more posterior parts of the MPFC are associated with the understanding of intentions inferred from physical cues (yellow) 23

Fig. 2.1: Example of emotion attribution based on a fulfilled intention (left) and an unfulfilled intention (right). Pictures were consecutively presented with intermediate fixation periods varying in time intervals. Functional analysis focused on the emotion attribution stimuli (picture 3; Study I) 29

Fig. 2.2: Example of a reality judgement trial. Pictures were consecutively presented with intermediate fixation periods varying in time intervals. Functional analysis focused on the reality processing stimuli (picture 3; Study I) 30

Fig. 3.1: Main effect of the factor intention-outcome-relation. Results were obtained during the fMRI session. Mean emotion attribution scores (+/-1 SE) in the intention fulfilled (light grey) compared to the intention unfulfilled emotion attribution condition (dark grey; Study I) 34

Fig. 3.2: Main effect of the factor intention-outcome-relation. Results were obtained during the rating task. Mean emotion attribution scores (+/-1 SE; 1 = not at all; 5 = very strong) in the intention fulfilled (light grey) compared to the intention unfulfilled emotion attribution condition (dark grey; Study I) 36

Fig. 3.3: (A) Functional changes in the amplitude of the HRF in the medial pre-SMA (BA6) associated with emotion attribution. (B) BA6 showed a significant signal increase associated with emotion attribution based on both an unfulfilled (EmoAtt-IntUnful) and fulfilled intention (EmoAtt-IntFul), compared to reality judgement (Non-Ment). HRF, hemodynamic response function; BA, Brodmann's area (Study I) 39

Fig. 3.4: (A) Functional changes in the amplitude of the HRF in the right dorsolateral prefrontal cortex (BA9) associated with emotion attribution. (B) BA9 showed a significant signal increase associated with emotion attribution based on an unfulfilled intention (EmoAtt-IntUnful) compared to reality judgement (Non-Ment). HRF, hemodynamic response function; BA, Brodmann's area (Study I) 40

Appendix A

Fig. 3.5: (A) Functional changes in the amplitude of the HRF in the left ventrolateral prefrontal cortex (BA47) associated with emotion attribution. (B) BA47 showed a significant signal increase associated with emotion attribution based on a an unfulfilled intention (EmoAtt-IntUnful) compared to reality judgement (Non-Ment). HRF, hemodynamic response function; BA, Brodmann's area (Study I) 41

Fig. 3.6: (A) Functional changes in the amplitude of the HRF in the orbital part of the paracingulate cortex (BA32) associated with emotion attribution. (B) BA32 showed a significant signal decrease in the intention unfulfilled condition (EmoAtt-IntUnful) compared to the intention fulfilled condition (EmoAtt-IntFul) Further, reality judgements (Non-Ment) were associated with a significant activity increase compared to both emotion attribution conditions. HRF, hemodynamic response function; BA, Brodmann's area (Study I) 42

Fig. 6.1: Example of emotions inferred from a fulfilled neutral intention (left) and an unfulfilled neutral intention (right). Pictures were consecutively presented with intermediate fixation periods varying in time intervals. Functional analysis focused on the emotion attribution stimuli (picture 3; Study II) 66

Fig. 6.2: Example of emotions inferred from a fulfilled immoral intention (left) and an unfulfilled immoral intention (right). Pictures were consecutively presented with intermediate fixation periods varying in time intervals. Functional analysis focused on the emotion attribution stimuli (picture 3; Study II) 67

Fig. 6.3: Example of a reality judgement trial. Pictures were consecutively presented with intermediate fixation periods varying in time intervals. Functional analysis focused on the reality processing stimuli (picture 3; Study II) 68

Fig. 7.1: Mean emotion attribution scores (+/- 1 SE) obtained during the fMRI session. Intention by intention-outcome-relation interaction effects were observed for positive (A) and negative (B) emotions (Study II) 75

Fig. 7.2: Main effects of the factors intention-outcome relation (A) and intention (B) in the rating task. Rating scores range from 1 (not at all) to 5 (very strong, Study II) 77

Fig. 7.3: Main effects of intention in the rating task for embarrassment (A) and sadness (B). Rating scores range from 1 (not at all) to 5 (very strong, Study II) 78

Fig. 7.4: Intention by intention-outcome relation interaction effects in the rating task. Rating scores range from 1 (not at all) to 5 (very strong, Study II) 79

Fig. 7.5: (A) Functional changes in the amplitude of the HRF in the medial pre-supplementary motor area (BA 6) associated with an intention by intention-outcome-relation interaction effect. (B) Post-hoc t-tests showed an activity increase for fulfilled immoral compared to fulfilled neutral intentions. HRF, hemodynamic response function; BA, Brodmann's areas are approximate (Study II) 88

Fig. 7.6: (A) Functional changes in the amplitude of the HRF in the left ventrolateral prefrontal cortex (BA 47) associated with an intention by intention-outcome-relation interaction effect. (B) Post-hoc t-tests showed an activity increase for fulfilled immoral compared to fulfilled neutral intentions. HRF, hemodynamic response function; BA, Brodmann's areas are approximate (Study II) 89

Fig. 7.7: (A) Functional changes in the amplitude of the HRF in the right ventrolateral prefrontal cortex (BA 45) associated with an intention by intention-outcome-relation interaction effect. (B) Post-hoc t-tests showed an activity increase for fulfilled immoral compared to fulfilled neutral intentions. HRF, hemodynamic response function; BA, Brodmann's areas are approximate (Study II) 90

Index of Tables

Tab. 3.1: Mean emotion attribution scores of the fMRI session for the intention fulfilled and intention unfulfilled emotion attribution condition (Study I) 33

Tab. 3.2: Mean emotion attribution scores of the rating task for the intention fulfilled and intention unfulfilled emotion attribution condition (Study I) 35

Tab. 3.3: Brain regions showing significant functional signal changes associated with emotion attribution (Study I) 38

Tab. 7.1: Mean emotion attribution scores of the fMRI session in the intention and in the intention-outcome-relation condition (Study II) 74

Tab. 7.2: Mean emotion attribution scores of the fMRI session dependent on the factor intention (neutral intention, immoral intention) and intention-outcome-relation (match: intention fulfilled, mismatch: intention unfulfilled; Study II) 74

Tab. 7.3: Mean emotion attribution scores of the rating task in the intention and in the intention-outcome-relation condition (Study II) 80

Tab. 7.4: Mean emotion attribution scores of the rating task dependent on the factors intention (neutral intention, immoral intention) and intention-outcome-relation (match: intention fulfilled, mismatch: intention unfulfilled; Study II) 80

Tab. 7.5: ANOVA of the emotion attribution results from the rating task (Study II) 81

Tab. 7.6: Post-hoc t-test results on the rating task to further analyse intention by intention-outcome-relation interaction effects (Study II) 82

Tab. 7.7: Brain regions showing significant functional signal changes associated with emotion attribution (Study II) 84

Tab. 7.8: Brain regions showing significant functional signal changes associated with the main effect of intention (Study II) 85

Tab. 7.9: Brain regions showing significant functional signal changes associated with intention by intention-outcome relation interaction effects (Study II) 86

Tab. 7.10: Post-hoc *t*-test results in brain regions showing significant functional signal changes associated with the intention by intention-outcome-relation interaction (Study II) 87

APPENDIX B

EXAMPLE OF THE RATING MATERIAL

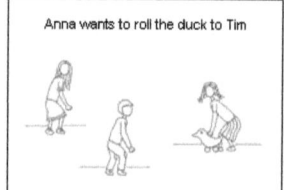
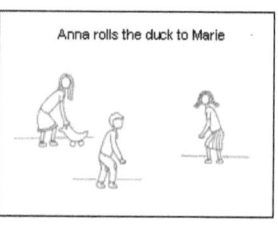
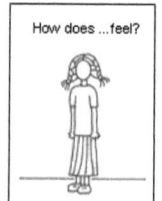

	not at all			very strong	
...neutral	1	2	3	4	5
...sad	1	2	3	4	5
...happy	1	2	3	4	5
...embarrassed	1	2	3	4	5
...surprised	1	2	3	4	5
...angry	1	2	3	4	5

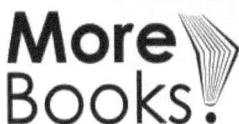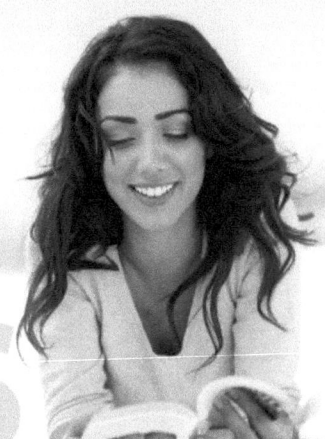

I want morebooks!

Buy your books fast and straightforward online - at one of world's fastest growing online book stores! Environmentally sound due to Print-on-Demand technologies.

Buy your books online at
www.morebooks.shop

Kaufen Sie Ihre Bücher schnell und unkompliziert online – auf einer der am schnellsten wachsenden Buchhandelsplattformen weltweit! Dank Print-On-Demand umwelt- und ressourcenschonend produziert.

Bücher schneller online kaufen
www.morebooks.shop

KS OmniScriptum Publishing
Brivibas gatve 197
LV-1039 Riga, Latvia
Telefax: +371 686 204 55

info@omniscriptum.com
www.omniscriptum.com

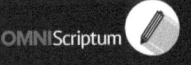

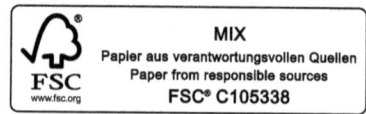

Printed by Books on Demand GmbH, Norderstedt / Germany